ULTRA-R
INTO RETIREMENT

OTHER TITLES BY PETER MCMANNERS
FOR SUSTA PRESS INCLUDE:

Face Up to Climate Change
ISBN: 978-0-9557369-4-0 (PB)

There should be no need for this book. We should have faced up to climate change decades ago. But we didn't, and now the world faces a crisis.

Climate change is a clear and present danger to society, and the current attempts at international climate policy are woefully inadequate. Breaking the cycle of failure requires careful examination of the cause. This book does that and proposes a pragmatic and practical alternative, how to cure fossil-fuel addiction and back off from cooking the planet.

Resilient Economics
ISBN: 978-0-9557369-6-4 (HB)

In good times, growth and profits are welcome, but in bad times, we need resilience, and resilience cannot be spirited up overnight.

The adoption of resilient economics should allow an economic system to evolve that is stable by default. The next crisis could be any number of issues, some very closely aligned with the economy and others related to health and environment, or something else entirely. A truly resilient economy should be able to weather any crisis and bounce back when it abates.

We need to recalibrate economics to regain its place as a solid and respected discipline at the heart of policymaking. Resilient economics can do this. It provides a framework that moves away from focussing on expansion and growth, to focussing on security, stability, and sustainability.

ABOUT THE AUTHOR

Dr Peter McManners is an author, consultant, and Visiting Fellow of Henley Business School. As an environmentalist, he has written many books about how to reshape the economy to be kinder to our planet. In his work as a Fellow, he leads a module on sustainability, arguing for fundamental change to how we think about economics and how to shape its application. He spends his leisure time off-road ultra-running, a passion of his that gives him ample time to reflect on these concepts.

ULTRA-RUNNING INTO RETIREMENT

PETER McMANNERS

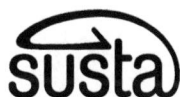

susta

SUSTA PRESS

12 Horseshoe Road, Pangbourne, Reading,
Berkshire RG8 7JQ, UK

Susta Limited is UK registered company
www.susta.co.uk

First published in Great Britain 2025
Copyright © Peter McManners, 2025

Peter McManners has asserted his right under the Copyright,
Designs and Patents Act, 1988, to be identified as Author of this work

A catalogue record for this book is available from the British Library

ISBN: PB: 978-0-9557369-9-5;
EBOOK: 978-1-0684587-0-5

Copyedited by Lisa Carden
Proofread by Eden Phillips Harrington
Project managed by Alysoun Owen Consulting Ltd.
Typeset by Catherine Lutman Design

Disclaimer: Peter McManners is not a medical doctor. The content of this book is
intended for informational and educational purposes only based on his own personal
experiences; it is not for the purpose of rendering medical advice. It is not intended
to substitute for professional medical advice, diagnosis or treatment.

CONTENTS

PREFACE

Retirement is often regarded as a time to wind down and enjoy leisurely activities. You can spend your time reflecting on memories of your life and take an interest, as an observer, in what the younger generation are doing. That is fine, but if this is *all* you do, you are missing out. Retirement brings with it the spare time and freedom to do whatever you want, including pushing forward in new directions. Instead of facing the certainty of a predictable slow decline, you have the option of grasping the opportunity of a renewed appetite for life, a fresh start, a new pursuit without knowing where it might take you. For me, the challenge I took on was ultra-running. For this slow-burn version of extreme sport, age is not a barrier. There is no need to set high expectations, and better that you don't. Turbocharging retirement by participating in ultra-running works at whatever level suits you. Start slow, and I suggest stay slow, letting the distance be the challenge.

Stopping paid employment and drawing your pension should not mark the beginning of the end, but can be the start of relaunching your life to do things you may only have dreamed of. This can be so much more than ticking off items on a so-called 'bucket list'. Although appropriate for someone of any age who is terminally ill, to cram the remaining time with memories, old age is not an illness. Retirement provides the chance for a total reboot in a new direction. Your life can be reinvigorated by taking yourself completely outside your comfort zone. You cannot regain your youth but you can recapture a youthful attitude. Try it; give it a go; take a risk; these are what drive younger people and can also revive the old, for those who rise to the challenge.

Retirement is one of life's great transitions, just as monumental as leaving school, starting your first job or getting married. Each transition closes one chapter and opens a new one. At the end of school, we leave the sheltered world of secondary education for the excitement of adult life. Getting married is to put behind the care-free life of a single person to take on the responsibility of building a family. Retirement means shrugging off the discipline of work and gaining the freedom to do whatever you want, whenever you want, however you want. Many retired people become slaves to the belief that retirement is the beginning of the end, a time to gently wind down mentally and physically. I oppose that attitude, arguing that retirement should be about taking on new challenges.

As I approached retirement, I was held back by stereotypical ideas of what it should comprise. I was sorely lacking ambition, a weakness which I am pleased to report I have now overcome. Initially, all I was looking for was one last big adventure whilst I still had strength and vitality. Like many others my age, I had fallen into the trap of believing that decline is inevitable. From this negative mindset I decided I should do something memorable, whilst I still could. During the process of pursuing what I believed would be my one last big adventure, I discovered how wrong this attitude was.

Planning my concluding escapade, I mulled over a few possibilities. The challenge which stood out above the other ideas was a race that had always fascinated me as something special, the Marathon des Sables (MDS). This week-long race across the Sahara requires runners to carry almost everything they need, including food for the entire week. The only item provided by the race organizers is water; otherwise, you need to be totally self-sufficient. I had dreamed of doing it but there was never time, or with a family to support too great a risk, or any number of other excuses not to chase this particular dream. Thinking about it, these excuses no longer applied. I had the time, and as for risk, this now applied only to me; my adult family would do just fine without me. The more I thought about it, the more I became convinced that this would be a suitable challenge for my final escapade, before bowing out.

I admit that my starting point in this quest was inherently negative. Wanting 'one last big adventure whilst I still had strength and vitality' turned out to be completely wrong. Retirement should have nothing to do with 'bowing out'. I discovered through the process of preparing for the MDS, competing in it, and then following it with yet tougher ultra-running challenges, that I was setting myself up for a better life. Rather than this being my final performance, this was the opening act of a new phase of life. Sit around doing nothing and we can be certain of following the standard script of slowing down, entering a care home, and finally expiring in a hospital bed. I don't want such certainty of outcome. I want the lottery of living life full-on until my number comes up. In this way, we will not know in advance how the story of our life ends – and better that we don't.

The training and preparations needed to be able to run across the desert gave me a new focus which consumed my attention for about eighteen months. I found the event to be even tougher than I had imagined, completing it soon after my sixtieth birthday. What I had not expected was how this would fire up inside me a passion for ultra-running. It is now in my blood, providing the context for staying fit and active for as long as I shall live. Ultra-running can ensure that the final phase of life is about quality of life rather than longevity.

By writing about my conversion to ultra-running, I hope that I can inspire others to thrive into old age, in whatever manner suits them. Factually, we all know that retirement is the final stage of life; that means it should be lived without compromise to extract the very best from the time remaining.

CHAPTER 1

REBEL AGAINST AGEISM

There is nothing sensible about ultra-running.

Society pressurizes older people to conform to a stereotype of retired bliss, coddled, cared for and protected. There are benefits that come with this paternal approach, such as a free bus pass, discounted travel and cheaper tickets for entertainment. Take advantage of these by all means but don't feel compelled to comply with what others might expect in the way you behave. The highlights of a retirement week could be coffee in a day centre; a game of bingo; or 'silver screenings' during the day when cinemas are otherwise empty. If this appeals to you, that is your choice, but I believe that there should be much more to retirement. Rebel against ageism by chasing your dreams, taking risks and exploiting the freedoms that retirement offers. The direction I have taken, and that I champion in this book, is to take up ultra-running. This is certainly not expected behaviour, and likely to attract well-meant but negative advice to stop being so silly and to be sensible instead. Such counsel is both wrong and right. It is wrong to regard ultra-running as silly as it helps you to remain fit, active, and happy into old age. It is right in that ultra-running is not sensible, but that should not rule it out. As you retire and escape the responsibilities that working-age adults endure, there is no need to be sensible. Instead of accepting slow terminal decline, embrace the concept of running right up until your final day. True, the extremes of ultra-running might ultimately become the cause of your demise, but I can't think of a better way to exit. Live life fully, without compromise, to really enjoy the final lap.

Ultra-running is defined as any distance longer than a marathon, but it can be much further. Putting on running shoes and lining up on the start line when the finish is 100 miles away, most sensible people would regard as bonkers. It is evidently a ridiculous thing to do, especially given that mental anguish and physical pain are an integral part of the experience. Why anyone would inflict this on themselves, by choice, is weird. It is even weirder to recommend that people take up ultra-running on retirement and continue into old age. Why do something so completely daft, illogical, crazy, even stupid? Yet I joined in the madness of ultra-running, and it helped me to turn back the years and bring retirement alive with a new sense of purpose.

Anyone, at any age, can change the direction of their life, but there is one inescapable truth. The truth is that it will end, some place, some time, in some way. Entering the last chapter of life is not the time to focus on delaying the inevitable by careful, safe and sheltered living. There is more to life than surviving for longer; it must be about living, really living, and accepting that this carries risk.

How crazy it is that young people with their whole lives ahead of them take extraordinary risks, whilst us oldsters tend to take extra care. This is the wrong way around. It is the young who should take care and the old who should go for it. That is not to say that an Formula 1 driver can be a pensioner. They would not have the speed of reaction required, but when there is a crash, in terms of loss of life, it would be better that someone from my generation was in the wreckage. The loss to family and society of the old departing is less, and arguably even a saving of resources better expended on training and educating the next generation. Venerating the old is good; listening to their advice and drawing on their experience and knowledge makes sense. Wrapping them in cotton wool and keeping them breathing long after senility sets in, does not. Surviving, defined as not yet being dead, is not living. I don't want to survive; I want to live.

Through middle age, the health and vitality of youth tends to drop away. Without taking remedial action, this slowdown will gather pace as part of the natural ageing process. This can be accepted and embraced for the freedom it gives. The freedom not to give a damn. That is what some people look forward to. This version of ageing can be enjoyed if your idea of living well is to do bugger all. I observe young people who have already given up on active health and rely on their youth to keep them in some sort of shape. This works in their twenties and perhaps thirties but someone reaching the age of forty without an active and healthy lifestyle is likely already to be on the path to decline. Worsening health is the direct consequence but correlated with this, there is often a decline in happiness and perhaps libido. By the age of fifty, some people are firmly entrenched on a downward trajectory. Sadly, that was me.

For more people than it should, life beyond sixty years of age enters a twilight zone. I admit that this was where I was heading, until I discovered that there is an elixir of youth, much better than statins, beta blockers and pills for high blood pressure. Adding ultra-running to this medicine chest can reverse the direction of travel. Instead of entering a downward spiral of failing health, you can choose to use the free time that retirement brings to increase physical activity. To make this choice, you accept that a light burning bright can burn itself out. It is possible to feel healthy and happy right up until the lights go out. In this way we do not just survive slow decline but remain active until our final day. Die healthy, die happy, die with your running shoes on.

Becoming an ultra-runner has opened a new perspective on retirement full of challenge and interest. Where it takes me, I do not know; if I am honest, I don't much care. The journey is just great.

The pinnacle of ultra-trail running is the Ultra Trail du Mont Blanc, known as the UTMB®. This race was definitely not on my retirement agenda, and I hesitate to recommend it to anyone of any age, but amongst ultra-runners it is special – and completely crazy. The route circumnavigates around the highest mountain in the Alps, connecting up by a number of mountain paths travelling through three countries: France, Switzerland and Italy. If you have hiked in this area, you know how beautiful the scenery is and how steep and rugged the paths are. Such a route could be a wonderful extended outdoor holiday: hiking each day; recovering each evening; and then repeat, to return to where you started perhaps ten days later. Ultra-runners have a different approach. The UTMB starts in the mountain town of Chamonix and arrives back where it began two days and two nights later, as one continuous race, without a break. The dedication, drive and pure grit of these runners seems almost beyond comprehension. It is something I would not have contemplated, either as a young man when I would not have had the mental discipline, nor as an old man slowing down with age. As I went through my initiation into ultra-running I became fascinated by the possibility of doing the UTMB, but I never thought I would actually enter it. That moment of complete madness did arrive eventually, but I am getting ahead of myself. How my attempt at the UTMB panned out can wait until later.

Before taking the plunge into ultra-running, I found myself approaching my sixtieth birthday, with old age just around the corner. Of course, old age is relative. 'Old' seems always to be a least ten years into the future. As a veteran runner aged forty, fifty seemed old. When I reached fifty, sixty looked old. When approaching sixty, I still felt young, observing people of seventy as old. Now, at the time of writing, well into my seventh decade, I still feel young and I have started considering how to mark my seventieth birthday. Eighty years of age seems old for sure, but experience tells me that when I reach that milestone, my perception of old will shift to ninety. That is if my body holds out long enough to reach these milestones.

The perspective at the heart of this book is not to accept age as a barrier. I know I cannot prevent *looking* older as the years tick by, but that does not need to degrade my enthusiasm for an active life. As we drive through life's journey, if we take our foot off the accelerator and pull over, it is possible to reflect and look around but, being stationary, no new experiences come into view. To continue to enjoy driving along the road requires you to keep your foot on the accelerator with a forward gaze to what adventures may lie on the road ahead. That does not prevent glancing in the rear-view mirror from time to time, though.

Reflecting back to my time as a young man, I dabbled in a number of sports. One of these was triathlon, which consists of swimming, cycling and a run. In the 1980s, this was an emerging new sport and an acquaintance, knowing I could both cycle and run, suggested I give it a try. In hindsight, I suspect that he might have been kidding and the suggestion was not intended as a serious proposal. Or, perhaps, he was not aware just how weak a swimmer I was, and assumed I was competent in the water. For me, the triathlon was a completely daft idea – perhaps as daft as taking up ultra-running in my sixties.

In the give-it-a-go mentality typical of young people, which I am pleased to write I still retain, I entered the British Long Course Triathlon Championships. This was quite literally jumping in at the deep end, and not a good choice for my first triathlon race. The race started with a 2 km swim. I observed other competitors wearing one-piece triathlon racing suits. I had a one-piece cycling time trial suit which looked similar, so I wore it. This turned out to be a bad choice. The tight Lycra suit had a well-padded chamois leather crotch, great for cycling, but not for swimming. The chamois leather became sodden and heavy, and the suit became baggy and filled with water. The drag from my inappropriate clothes made my basic breaststroke even slower. I finished the swim second to last. Behind me was one old man, old in my terms back then but probably only as old as I am now. As this new sport was so new, he must have taken it up in retirement, so a good example of the lifestyle championed in this book.

Following my ignominious start, I spent the bike race segment overtaking a lot of competitors. It was the same on the run, blasting out my best pace for the half marathon. My final position was towards the middle of the pack. I enjoyed my first stab at the triathlon so much that I joined my local triathlon club in order to learn to swim. I could already swim, in terms of staying afloat and not drowning, but my feeble breaststroke was, to triathletes, laughable. I started in the slowest lane in the pool on my first training night. The swim coach asked me to swim a couple of lengths freestyle to show my standard. I asked if that was nonstop, as I hadn't learnt the breathing technique required for freestyle. She gave me a look as if to say 'are you serious?'. Her initial feedback on my first triathlon swim training session was to question whether triathlon was the sport for me. More positively, she said that there was plenty of room for improvement. Over the next two years, I did learn to breathe correctly and was steadily promoted up the lanes as my fitness and technique improved; I ended up swimming in the fastest lane. This was a triumph of determination over ability. I was never going to be one of the fastest triathletes, as I had come to race swimming as an adult. I hadn't learnt the fast fluid style of a good swimmer. I swam with too much splashing and not enough of the technique needed to be able to slip through the water at speed. Even so, I became fast enough to compete at international level as an amateur age-group competitor. When young, these are challenges to relish, and your body can handle the hard training required.

Like many young triathletes, I was somewhat dismissive of the men in the senior age categories who turned up at world championship races, trying to shave off a few minutes by purchasing top-end expensive bikes. Youthful aspiring athletes, squeezing the fastest pace out of the best bike they could afford, would look on with envy at these top-notch bikes being ridden relatively slowly. That observation was useful as I became one of those older men. I kept the same racing bike throughout my time racing triathlon, upgrading only with better wheels. My race bike was battered, scratched and looked old, but I took pride in riding it at a speed that defied its appearance.

One positive memory from my triathlon racing days is drawn from a low-key race in the build-up to one of the world championship events. My memory of exactly where has faded but it was held on the coast with the start and finish on the beach. At this small local triathlon, I was on the results list as a winner of one of the minor places. I waited around for the prize-giving, soaking up the sun and lounging on the beach. The prize-giving was delayed to allow the winner of the over-eighty age category the time to complete the event. Like many competitors in this informal event, he was wearing only swimming trunks and running shoes as he shuffled over the line. It reminded me that when you reach eighty, you cannot hide your age. The loose wrinkled skin is a fact of old age. In this case, the impression was reinforced by his choice of swimming costume which was large, loose and faded by the sun. Speedos they were not. I did not then identify with him, but I was impressed by his determination and admired his I-do-not-care-what-you-think attitude. He was a winner in his own terms and fully deserved the applause as he finished. Even though, as the only entrant in his age group, the winner's prize required only that he finish. My younger self was not thinking that this was going to be me half-a-century hence.

As I reached 58¾, I started thinking about a way to mark my sixtieth birthday. I am not someone who likes being the centre of attention at a party, so a large gathering was not what I was looking for. The occasion would have to be memorable and involve doing something special and challenging.

For my fiftieth, I had travelled to the town of Lahti in southern Finland and skied 50 km cross country stopping to meet one expatriate friend who lived in Finland for lunch halfway. The café selected was located beneath the ski jump tower in the winter sports complex. The walls were covered with posters of previous ski events and I could imagine being a great cross-country skier. This was a long way short of the truth, but I was free to embrace such a dream for the day. Leaving the warm sanctuary of the café after lunch to complete the challenge took a bit of determination but I had found the day fulfilling.

For my sixtieth, I considered getting back on cross-county skis to ski 60 km, but that would have been too similar. I was feeling the sands of time slip by and wanted something new and challenging. As I contemplated my options, I thought about what I might be capable of. Up to this point in my life, I had always considered myself fit and able to have a go at just about anything. I realized that that was no longer so. My strength was waning, there were signs of flabbiness around my waist, and I was now prone to injury if running longer distances, particularly if this was over rough terrain. My body was clearly winding down. The advice I was getting was to stop running to save my knees. I hear this often in conversation with people my age, that knees should be conserved through stopping the pounding. I was also told that middle-age spread is normal and even overheard a comment that fat around the midriff is inevitable and cannot be avoided. From this perspective, perhaps I needed a hiking challenge, with lunch in the pub, and the number of a taxi firm in my pocket in case lunch were to prove too intoxicating.

'No!,' I thought. Despite the reality of the numbers, I do not feel old. I do not want to slow down. I do not want to be offered a seat on trains and buses by polite and well-meaning young people. Sod them. Their efforts should be employed directed at pensioners – ignoring the fact that I was not far off pensionable age myself. I decided that I would not conform to the behaviours stereotypical of people my age.

I was thinking about something challenging, something outside my comfort zone, something about which I could not be sure of achieving. A challenge is only a challenge where failure is possible. One of the annoyances of the modern social-media age is the presentation of things that are easy, as challenges. People seek publicity and perhaps sponsorship for things they would find easy – or which they would want to do in any case. Why sponsor someone to have fun? Tandem parachuting falls into this category. Nothing to be done except go along for the ride with the expert parachutists in control and pulling the strings. Jumping out of a plane alone with your own parachute would be worth sponsoring. That scares the crap out of you, as I know only too well from my early career in the military. It is especially fear-inducing when at low-level, at night, into an unfamiliar drop zone. For a running example, consider a regular 5 km park runner, seeking sponsorship to run 10 km. To my mind, that would be to extort money by false pretences. A real challenge for such a person might be to run a marathon. That would be a decent reason to seek sponsorship money for a charity. Challenging should mean challenging, with the outcome not preordained.

The 100 miles of the UTMB, non-stop through mountainous terrain, certainly does count as challenging. This mammoth race had not been in the frame for my sixtieth birthday challenge. As someone from outside the ultra-running community, I had not even heard of it. If this race had been brought to my attention, I would have rejected it as a challenge too far. The race which I *had* heard about, and which I started to consider, was the race with a fearsome reputation, the legendary MDS. As noted above, this week-long race across the Sahara requires that you carry on your back everything you need, including food, with water resupply the only exception. It was established in 1986 and has earned the strap line 'the toughest foot race on Earth'. I was happy to go along with this claim, even though I subsequently discovered that there are even tougher and longer events. The idea of doing the 'toughest foot race on Earth' to mark my sixtieth seemed like suitably challenging. It fitted the criteria that success should not be a given; there needed to be real doubt about whether it could be done. My doubts were very real, but I put them aside, avoiding thinking too much about what it would require of me and more about the feeling if indeed I could finish.

The MDS is not a sensible choice for a first ultramarathon, but I did not intend this to be the start of a passion for ultra-running. This was to be a one-off event, simply one last blast before bowing out on a high and accepting old age as fact. Ultra-running had never appealed to me. Running slowly seemed silly when you could enter shorter races and run fast – by whatever metric fits your ability. My longest race before my decision to enter the MDS had been the marathon. Plenty long enough to be a real test, with sufficient potential to stress the body to the limit of what I thought was possible whilst wearing running shoes. I was to discover that I was wrong; the marathon is nothing compared with what ultra-running has to offer.

To run slowly is easy. The first twenty minutes is just a warm-up. The first hour is a breeze. The first five hours goes by without drama. The race then starts. During the next five hours, it starts to get uncomfortable. The next thirty hours becomes painful in a way that cannot be described and can be understood only by experiencing it. Every five-minute section of an ultra-run is easy. It is when many hundreds of these are put back-to-back that it becomes hard. This is where the psychology clicks in. It is always possible to run another five minutes, so you remain in that mindset of 'just another five minutes'. This mental technique rescued me in the Alps during a storm at night, on a steep climb with thick mud interspersed with rocks. I moved off to the side of the track, sat on a rock; switched off my head torch so no one would observe my failure, and put my head in my hands. I felt that I could not take another step. I was cold and getting colder; I could have stopped right there and slipped away into quiet oblivion. In a sense, what a way to go. It would have been a better conclusion to life than bed-ridden in a care home for the elderly. But self-preservation is a powerful instinct. I rummaged in my pocket for a piece of chocolate, got up and did another five minutes, and another, and another, until the first light of dawn switched my mood from negative to positive. That experience was to be logged later when I finally did enter the seemingly impossible UTMB; but first was the MDS.

The experience of doing the MDS, and the training leading up to it, changed my outlook. Slow running, such as jogging a few km, is indeed easy. Ultra-running is different. It is masochistic slow torture to be savoured and enjoyed. Sleep deprivation only sharpens the out-of-body experience as your mind escapes to another place. Whatever troubles and concerns you may have in your life are incinerated in a furnace of hurt.

There is no logical reason to take up ultra-running, particularly in retirement. However, many of the best, most enjoyable aspects of life do not conform to such simple logic. We do stuff simply because it is fun. The same applies to ultra-running: do it because you can; do it because it makes you feel good (even if only after you have stopped); do it to turn back time and defy the ageing process.

CHAPTER 2

ULTRA-RUN FOR FUN

Regular running lifts your mood
and can be fun, provided you persevere.

In the normal flow of life, for an activity to be regarded as fun, it needs to provide an immediate positive hit. This might be a stroll amongst bluebells in spring sunshine, watching a good film, playing a game, socializing with friends, or any number of enjoyable pursuits. Set loose by the freedom of retirement, having fun can become a priority. Choosing an enjoyable activity translates into fun as soon as you start doing it. Ultra-running does not conform to this easy logic. It will not be fun until you have logged a good chunk of mileage to attune your body to running with ease. It is not intrinsically fun, and it is not easy to make it fun. Unless it is fun, it is unlikely to become a habit, especially in retirement when no-one is pressurizing you to do anything. So how do you progress from giving it a try to really enjoying it?

The key to making ultra-running fun is the approach you take. Regarding it as racing or competing won't work, particularly as you get older and slower. What was once an easy jog becomes your racing pace. Ultra-running in your twilight years should be about participating. Do not enter an ultramarathon to win, or to compete against anyone but yourself. The competition is to complete the event. The prize is to finish.

As we age, our tolerance of things we don't enjoy wanes. We are no longer bound by the duty of work or the responsibly of parenthood, things that steer us to do what should be done. When younger, we might have run because we are told it is good for us, because we enjoy a race, or because we look good in Lycra.

These three reasons do not require that it must be fun. None of these applies in older age. First, old people are not generally advised that running is good for them. Second, enjoying racing does not last because age inevitably slows us down and makes us uncompetitive (except against people our own age). Third, as for looking good in Lycra, I shall say no more. If running is not fun, older people shorn of expectation and responsibility are likely to take a simple approach to encouragement to run, which might be expressed as 'sod off'.

To make an activity feel like fun, there is a selection of tonics we can use including alcohol, nicotine or other substances. These can enhance our enjoyment and bring more fun into our lives, but at a cost to both the wallet and health. I suggest endorphins should be added to this list. These are produced by your body when you run, cost nothing and are positive for health. It is simple to grab a beer from the fridge or pour a glass of Chardonnay, sit and enjoy. It is almost as easy to put on running shoes and get out the door to enjoy the freedom of movement and filling your lungs with fresh air. It only works if you run regularly; if you run rarely, doing so is not likely to fill you with joy.

To pretend that running is enjoyable by default fools no one. Without working at making running fun, it never will be fun. If you don't run, perhaps have never run regularly, and don't have the passion to want to run, it is likely to be parked in your mind as punishment to be avoided. That is a shame, because getting into running through enduring the initial slog of training can take you to running Nirvana. That leads into a word of caution, as it can be the case that people who discover running later in life become zealots. Such overreaction can be counterproductive and lead to burn-out. To cement a life-long running habit, enthusiasm should be tempered by ensuring it remains fun.

In arguing that running can and should be fun, I accept that it is an acquired taste. As a boy, my first sip of beer tasted horrid, as the flavour of the hops met young taste buds. A little later in life, beer became a drink to enjoy. The same is true of running. If you don't run, or have not run recently, running feels heavy with jolting impact on the joints. It does not feel good and certainly is not fun. When you string together a long enough sequence of runs, you can acquire the taste for it. You start to get a spring in your legs that wasn't there before. Your mind and body work together to develop a smooth style that minimizes the risk of injury. This requires little conscious effort. It is allowing the body the circumstances to turn on instinctive actions. Humans have been running for thousands of years and the code is there in our DNA: it just needs to be activated.

Eventually, after many miles on numerous days, you seem almost to float over the ground, one leg landing after the other in sequence to provide smooth forward motion. Watching fast runners is to see poetry in motion. Slow running can also be smooth and easy if you do enough of it. You can graduate from an awkward slow plod to an enjoyable slow cruise. When you reach this level, your mind is set free to enjoy moving through your own efficient effort. Your running will not be effortless, but slow and relaxed low-level exertion, which can be sustained almost indefinitely when you have cracked the code.

There are barriers to overcome in the process of making running fun. One of these is the need to be strong and resilient. When I started ultra-running, it was well into middle age, and I had allowed the ageing process to take hold. Each year I had become weaker, slowly degenerating through laziness without noticing how a series of imperceptible changes were adding up to a weak and flabby body. In my mind I was still an athlete, but the reality was different. As I started to redress this neglect through running more, a series of injuries followed. That was depressing and definitely not fun. I discovered through bitter experience that if your only exercise is to run, you get injured. Running requires strength and resilience, but the conundrum is that it does not nurture either of them. Running smoothly and effortlessly doesn't cause injury; injuries happen when there is an unexpected event like slipping, sliding, tripping or falling. This is where you need strength throughout your body to be able to brace and halt the slide, recover from the trip or land safely as you hit the ground. The action of running does not give your body the strength to deal with these occasional incidents. This means strength-building exercises must go alongside running, to keep you free of injury and set up the possibility that you will embrace ultra-running as fun. These should also be fun, so they are appealing, rather than regarded as a chore. This is where I really struggle. One approach is to attend classes where you are told what to do and perhaps enjoy the social interaction. Another might be to go online for inspiration and support. It might be that exercising to music is your thing, although it doesn't float my boat. The solution that works for me is to establish resilience-building exercises as a habit that is consistent and just as routine as brushing my teeth. You don't reflect on whether brushing your teeth is fun or not. The activity does not rise up your conscious hierarchy to consider whether it is enjoyable.

The habits I have in place are a set of exercises each morning and evening. My routine never changes, both in terms of the exercises and the number of repetitions. This fixed routine has two benefits. First, it requires no conscious thought. I wake up, get out of bed, do my exercises and only then think about what I will do for the rest of the day. Second, the identical exercise set has now been part of my daily routine ever since my sixtieth birthday. It was a challenging workout for the middle-aged body

I had when I started, but now I am stronger and find the exercise set quite easy. That said, I don't increase the number or severity of the exercises for fear of escalating to the point where I give up. My thinking is that each day I can do the same easy routine, this year, next year, into my seventies, eighties and perhaps even nineties – if I keep the spark of life that long. There should be no reason why, if I can do the exercises one day, that I cannot repeat the next. This could continue for the rest of my life (unless major illness intrudes). It is an unswerving, unchanging, non-negotiable daily habit.

Simple daily body exercises may not be fun in themselves but when the habit has become deeply engrained, they occupy your physical body for a short time each morning and evening. As you do them, your mind it is free to reflect forward on the day ahead for morning exercises, or for evening exercise to reflect back on the past day. Physically easy and mentally relaxing turns out to be a perfect combination. This habit nurtures physical resilience, but you also need strength. That is where time in the gym comes in.

The gym has endless opportunities for variety and fun. I have happy memories from my younger days of lifting weights in time with reggae music as part of a group of active young people. The focus was on the music and keeping to the rhythm of the beat, making a potentially repetitive routine boisterous enjoyment. Each person should find their own version of fun in the gym but it's vital that you do. For older people, the gym helps you to push back against the ageing process. Getting weaker with age is programmed into our body clocks. The clock can be paused, or even reversed, through weight training. Stressing our bodies in this way causes microdamage to the muscles initiating the body's repair mechanism. As the ageing process leads to declining strength, another process is increasing it. With luck, one will balance out the other. It is not about becoming a muscle-bound weightlifter;

it is about keeping the strength we have and stopping the decline. On average, I go to the gym three days a week. The benefit is crystallized by the body repairing afterwards. So, to ensure full recovery I never do two days in the gym back-to-back. From one day to the next, you are unlikely to notice what the gym does for you, but over the months you will really feel the benefit. Like running, the occasional trip to the gym can feel like a chore, but once the gym has become a regular part of your life, you feel much stronger to take on whatever life might throw at you.

Returning the focus to running, regular running gives your life a boost, lifts your mood and can be fun. The body responds naturally to the demands you place on it. Ask nothing of it and you'll become weak and flabby; go running regularly and you become lean and toned. This is simple cause-and-effect. There is no need for dieting to maintain a healthy weight; if you run, the body is clever at keeping within a good running weight. The dietary advice that should be heeded concerns *what* you eat rather than how much you eat. Junk food is never healthy and to be avoided – this includes the empty calories in energy drinks. I am amazed that ordinary people succumb to the marketing hype for branded energy drinks aimed at encouraging their consumption during exercise. Although athletes at the top of their game and training hard over long sessions may need to ingest such pure fuel to be able to handle the heavy training load, for us mere mortals there is no need. The companies pedalling these unhealthy sugary drinks try to convince us otherwise, but don't be fooled. Sticking to water is better for you, more enjoyable, and allows you to look forward to proper food when you get home. When you run, there is no need to watch the calories. In fact, you should up your consumption, provided it is real nutritious food. Calorie counting is a fool's game; running works much better.

Choosing your route can be a large part of making running fun. When running has been established as a regular activity, your body will have naturally adopted a fluid and easy style. You can enjoy the simple pleasure of moving under your own power, blood pumping, joints moving and keeping bodily processes tip-top. An interesting and uplifting route completes an enjoyable package. You may be fortunate and live on the edge of a national park with hills and mountains accessible as soon as you leave your house. Even city dwellers should be able to put together a route that links up parks, canal towpaths and, in the absence of anything better, well-lit suburban streets with good walkways.

In retirement, you are free to choose time and place, making use of your free bus pass to go further afield. If you get bored with your regular routes, change them. For my part, liking simplicity, I repeat a standard set of my routes making maximum use of off-road paths and taking in available hills. I leave the house and get going without needing to think. I time my runs, but I avoid looking at my watch as I run. I no longer set targets or try to hold pace but do record the time after I get home just to see if the time matches how I feel. I am often surprised that what felt like an easy cruise was quite fast, not fast from a runner's perspective of course, but fast from *my* perspective.

To continue enjoy running into later life, do only the amount of running you find fun. This is where training plans have a chequered history. I have training plans and a training log, but the way I use them is not what running magazines generally recommend. An ambitious training plan that leads you to beat yourself up when you fail to complete it, is not part of making running fun. On the other hand, a training plan that focusses on ensuring you do not do too much, and limits how much you run, can work well.

There is plenty of advice to be found about training plans: some is good and some for older runners is exceedingly bad. Good advice is not to increase your weekly running mileage by more than 10 per cent week-on-week. Your body needs time to adapt and exceeding this can lead to injury. Your training log can ensure that you keep to this limitation. Bad advice is weekly mileage targets. Yes, log how far you run but don't become slave to total mileage targets. Professional runners set targets, which can seem huge. There is no point trying to emulate them. They do it because they have sponsors to please and medals they want to win. Whether or not it is fun does not enter the equation. Many fast successful athletes have come to see running as a day job from which they retire, meaning they miss out on the long-term benefits of making running fun into their retirement.

As a younger man, I used training plans in a different way, to serve a different purpose. I enjoyed racing and wanted to get faster. I would regard the plan as that which must be achieved. If I felt good on any particular day, I would add in another interval or tack on another few kilometres. Now that I am older, I have reversed this. The plan is useful to avoid thinking about what run I should do today. Look at the plan and just do it; but important psychologically I never doing more than is in the plan. The other training rule I have adopted is to always allow doing less. If you start running and it does not feel good, you feel tired, or in any way not enjoying it, stop and go home. Do make a start by getting out the door, but without the pressure of needing to complete the planned session. Mostly, once I am outside and have warmed into the run, I carry on as planned. The value to allowing less is that it emphasizes that running should be fun. If you fail to complete the plan more than once, don't see this as failure but rather an indication that the plan is wrong. Adjust the plan to fit what *is* fun and you will then be back on track.

It may seem odd to limit training when the aim is ultra-distance running. Simple logic would conclude that this requires an ultra amount of training. The problem with this is that this not likely to be fun and certainly not likely to engender continued enjoyment into old age. To participate in ultra-running events requires that you are able to run slowly. The main requirement is a mental attitude which gets you to the end. In training, my longest run does not exceed five hours. That could be a long morning, lining yourself up for a big lunch followed by an afternoon snooze. Ensure it stays fun by doing this no more than once a month, so you look forward to it with anticipation rather than trepidation. I am not sure which is the best aspect: the long run, the big feed or the siesta. As a package, it is just great.

To keep your monthly long run fun, you could try entering a low-key local marathon. Don't try to blitz a time, just cruise as if this was the first half of an ultramarathon to end slowly, feeling good.

Dressing appropriately is another part of the package of making running fun. Running clothes should be comfortable, keeping you warm, or cool, as required. Bright reflective colours are good so that you can be seen. For some people, the brand of running clothes they wear matters. For me, as long as it works, that is fine. One of my favourite items is a pair of Ron Hill tracksters that are over forty years old. They are frayed and looking their age, but fit like a second skin. Shoes are vital, of course, and it is not easy to find pairs that suit the exacting requirements of ultra-running. There is no alternative to trying several brands and models to find out what suits you. Price is not a good guide: my worst pair of running shoes were also my most expensive. I had suffered a stress fracture and wanted the very best shoes to prevent recurrence. In my mind I equated price with quality, and it led me astray. I bought a very expensive pair of shoes and hated them: they did not feel right. Later, I looked more closely at the marketing spiel and realized these shoes from a top brand were a fashion item to be worn to show off. I donated them to a charity shop within days of buying them. I am sure they will have been snapped up, but I hope their new owners were not intending to use them for running or, like me, they would have been disappointed. Marketing copy should not be used to choose shoes. It is better to observe what runners are actually wearing in ultra-running events. The final judgement is what feels right, does not cause blisters, and provides impact reduction cushioning without being spongy or too soft. A final obvious piece of advice is never to race in new shoes. Formula 1 drivers like to use new tyres; ultra-runners like well-proven shoes that have already gone a good distance.

Being kitted out appropriately for the weather is vital too. As the adage holds, there is no bad weather for running, just bad dressing. As a young man, my idea of an exhilarating run was to get out into the hills in bad weather dressed only in shorts and vest. I had to run fast to stay warm. The raw pleasure of being exposed to the elements while running fast over rough terrain was hard to beat. There was a sense of invulnerability overriding logical analysis. Coming a cropper could soon degenerate into hypothermia, though. Even experienced ultra-runners can descend into such stupidity. In 2021, a 62 mile ultramarathon race in Gansu province, China, was hit by severe weather including freezing rain, high winds and hail. Twenty-one runners died, including some of the runners in the leading pack. They had been wearing running shorts and vests, carrying the barest minimum according to the list of mandatory equipment, with gossamer-thin emergency clothes packed in micro backpacks. The items were chosen to satisfy spot race inspections, rather than effective mountain gear. The race organizers were prosecuted for ignoring extreme weather warnings, but the deceased runners were also at fault. It is important to take responsibility for your own safety and have what you need, which you have tested and know works. Layers are good, as are zips to open and close so that you can regulate temperature. I like to have pockets large enough for hat and gloves. You can wear these at the start of a long run and put them in your pockets when you are warm, with easy access should you need to stop for whatever reason. If you are somewhere remote, always carry a backpack containing (as the bare minimum): a light, warm, waterproof coat and a mobile phone. Do it because it is sensible, safe and gives peace of mind, not because of any rules that require it. Dress well to ensure your fun is not undermined by discomfort. Dress well to stay safe and have the peace of mind that you are safe whatever the weather throws at you.

A more controversial aspect of making running fun, which is peculiar to ultra-running, is to learn to enjoy pain. It might seem counterintuitive that pain and fun can be bedfellows. It certainly requires a degree of masochism. There will always be niggles and pains that should be noticed, as they are your body's way of talking to you. Your body is trying to tell you something, so listen; but the fact that you are hurting does not mean you have to stop. More on this is in the next chapter because pain and ultra-running are inseparable. If you set out to seek pain, that might indicate a mental health issue. To learn to enjoy the feeling of legs 50 km into a run is practical advice to develop the mental resilience for ultra-running. On one person's dashboard this might register as pain, but this is simply a feeling to embrace and not an indication of anything more serious.

To conclude this discussion about running for fun, if you are already a regular runner you will know that running *can* be fun. I hope that a few of the ideas here might help you to sustain that enjoyment into later life. If you are not a runner, I encourage you to try running regularly for at least one month. Less is not long enough to give your body time to adapt. Don't expect to enjoy the first month because if you are not a runner, running isn't fun. It is possible that injury may interrupt the month because people who don't run do not have the physical resilience of a runner. Provided you have not succumbed to injury, nor decided to quit before the month is up, I would be surprised if, at the end of the trial, if you had not perked up.

Running is fun, provided you are proactive in making it so.

CHAPTER 3

THE ENJOYMENT OF PAIN

'What painkillers do you use?'

This is the question I was asked by the race doctor at my medical check-up in the desert camp before starting the week-long race across the Sahara Desert.

The arrival into Morocco was on a flight into the small remote airport serving Ouarzazate, 200 km south-east of Marrakesh. The plane was chartered for the MDS so everyone on board was competing in the race. I was wearing my running shoes and carrying my racing backpack as hand luggage. Going to the trouble of entering and training for the MDS, I did not want to risk losing vital items if my luggage were to go astray. Many others did the same, all sharing the same concern. We should not have worried; the airport was a single runway and a small terminal building with few facilities, and ours seemed to be the only flight. One flight, one luggage belt, so little chance of confusion. Sets of steps on wheels were pushed across the tarmac to line up with the aeroplane's front and rear doors. When the aircraft doors opened, there was a blast of heat. It was like stepping into an oven as we walked down the steps onto the tarmac. This hot, dry and dusty location already felt like we were on the edge of the Sahara, which of course we were. We then boarded a fleet of chartered buses to be driven yet deeper into the desert until we arrived at the MDS camp. This is where the last trappings of everyday life were abandoned for a week of self-sufficiency in the desert.

On arrival in the camp, the most striking feature were the traditional Bedouin shelters erected in a wide circle. Aerial pictures of this huge and impressive tent circle in the desert are iconic of the MDS. There were eight of us allocated to Tent 119, all of us from the UK. We met for the first time on the bus but would get to know each other very well as the race progressed. There is nothing like sharing extreme toil and discomfort with others, especially where there is a complete lack of privacy, to build bonds of respect and friendship.

The MDS desert camp would move each day to a new location. Local workers would dismantle and reassemble it whilst we were running the day's stage. These were not tents in the way we would think of tents for camping. The shelters were large pieces of black hessian held aloft by wooden poles fashioned from pieces of gnarled tree branches of a variety of sizes and shapes. There were no sides to these shelters, with air flowing freely underneath, and nowhere for privacy. These were excellent protection from the sun but offered no defence against sandstorms – as we would discover later in the week.

In the tent, there was space for each of us to lie down, but not much more. This would be our night-time home for the next week, with the camp in a different place each night. The ground beneath was sometimes forgiving, and sleep relatively comfortable, and in other places stony hard.

The basic hessian shelter is all that the race provides; as I've explained already, everything else other than water had to be carried. A balance needed to be struck between comfort at night and the weight of the backpack carried through the day. The desert is relatively cold at night, so a sleeping bag was needed. My dream that we would be sleeping on soft sand was well adrift from reality, so it was fortunate that I had decided to carry a sleeping mat, cut down to the minimum size to give the upper body a degree of cushioning. My sleeping bag was a micro cocoon. This was all part of my efforts to get my backpack down to under 10 kg (including a week's food). Non-essential items were not included. Those that were needed were cut down to minimum weight. I included a pair of flip-flops to wear in camp but carefully cut off the bottom so they were half the thickness. Perhaps in doing this I had gone too far as there was little protection from sharp stones, but I had enjoyed the game of marginal weight reduction. A few grams less here and there all subtracted from the total load.

The first night in the desert was an easy introduction, with a simple meal provided by the race organizers. There was no need to dip into our race rations just yet. We got familiar with our tent buddies and introduced ourselves to the people in the tents on either side. Remember that these were simple hessian sun screens without walls, so not recognizable as a conventional tent. Our tent was an eclectic mix of different abilities and ages (I was the oldest by some way). I wondered who in our group would survive crossing the Sahara. The others might have been wondering whether the old man could make it. The first night gave us the chance to experience the magic of sleeping outside through a desert night without the pressure of ultra-running.

There was then a full day in camp before the race start, allowing us to get used to the spartan conditions of the desert. It was also the opportunity for the race organizers to ensure all runners were sufficiently prepared. There were several pre-race checks, for which we stood queuing in the sun. This was a warning to us of what was to come as the sun had a searing intensity. The sun was beating down on us and roasting our race backpacks that we were carrying for the check of the required mandatory equipment. When I opened mine, I came across the bar of dark chocolate I had packed to eat on the flight but had forgotten about. It was not just softened by the sun but had liquified and spread through the contents of my backpack. The kit inspector had a wry chuckle at my expense, exposing me as an amateur in the desert ultra fraternity. Throughout the week, the remnants of this sticky mess served as a reminder of my silly error.

Another check was whether you had packed enough food for a week. Again, a balance had to be struck between nutrition and the weight of the backpack. I carried the minimum calories specified in the race regulations. To minimize weight, I packed the most nutrition-dense food items I could find. I had one freeze-dried meal for each evening, some nuts and a selection of protein bars, making for a very hungry week in the desert. The final pre-race check was an interview with the race doctor.

People regularly die attempting the MDS. It is not widely advertised, and the statistics are not on the event website, but this is the reality. This is not the fault of the race organizers, but simply a consequence of the extreme nature of the event. The race organizers insist on several medical safeguards. For the compulsory medical check with the race doctor, I needed to produce a signed certificate from my own GP to declare I was medically fit to run. I also had to carry an ECG printout, which the race doctor could check for reassurance that my heart would be up to the challenge. It was during this interview with the race doctor that he asked, 'What painkillers do you use?'. He wanted to know what drugs I was carrying. I was surprised and a bit perplexed. On a personal level, I avoid medication, and in principle drugs should not be used in any sport. I answered, 'None, of course'. I found out later that painkillers are a standard item for many ultra-runners, using over-the-counter drugs such as aspirin, paracetamol or ibuprofen. Even more surprising to me was the insight that not only do runners carry such drugs, but some ultra-runners take them during the second half of an extreme ultra as routinely as they might snack on a food bar. To me, this is plain wrong. Painkillers are for extreme situations, which does not include the routine pain that always accompanies the ultra experience. This is to be accepted, and even enjoyed.

In an ultra-running race, it is normal to be completely and absolutely wiped out. This is not pain. This is simply chronic fatigue, which from the perspective of finishing must be faced down and endured. The approach I have just described is inherently negative. A positive perspective is to learn to embrace the out-of-body experience of extreme fatigue. Both perspectives relate to the same reality of a body that is hurting. Hurting isn't pain.

Sharp pain that is coming from a specific part of the body is sending a message. Listen to the message and decipher it. What has caused the pain and what can be done to alleviate it? If the cause is one that can be dealt with, then stop and deal with it. If the pain is in your feet, your socks might be out of place, your shoelaces too tight, or there could be a stone in your shoe. Fix the cause and carry on. With feet, blisters are always a risk. Once formed, they are not going away. They might be stabilized by adjusting your footwear, but the more likely outcome is that they get bigger, and wider, and then burst. This is not going to repair whilst the race is in progress. All you can expect is to keep it strapped up and clean, hoping that you don't get a deep secondary blister under the area of broken skin or, in longer races, an infection. When your feet have become one big, blistered mess, every foot landing is painful. Such constant pain becomes a distraction from just how tired you are. Ironically, if you embrace the pain of blisters, it masks the fatigue and carries you through to the end.

The question arises as to why it makes sense to push back against the body's natural warning mechanism. It would be logical to stop the activity causing the pain. If ultra-runners adopted this approach, sensible though it might be, it is doubtful that anyone would ever finish. Anyone who finishes an ultra-run claiming not to have experienced pain either has an exceptional running style that is smooth and easy on the body – or is lying. My running is certainly not of that standard, and I know that many ultra-runners are the same. At my first 100 mile ultra-run, you were allowed two drop bags, one available at halfway and the other to be waiting for you at the 80-mile aid station. Having started in the morning, it was dark when I arrived at that aid station, based in a village hall. I sat down with my reclaimed drop bag, completely knackered and at a very low ebb. I observed other runners with their drop bags; many of them pulled out what seemed like complete medical kits. They removed their shoes and socks, took a scalpel to remove the loose skin of broken blisters and then applied an antiseptic spray and taped up their feet, put their shoes back on and carried on. My feet were beacons of pain. Some miles before the aid station, I had felt the blisters on the soles of my feet, which had been sore and getting bigger, pop with a blast of intense pain. Although out of sight inside my running shoes, there was no doubt what had happened. I had had to adjust to a new and higher level of pain to carry on. In my drop bag, I had packed my favourite food bars, a fresh pair of socks and a couple of plasters, but no scalpel, antiseptic or medical tape. Without the means to copy the more experienced runners, I decided to leave my shoes on. I had not wanted to see just how bad the damage was, without the means to doing anything much about it. I told myself that it could not be anything serious, just peripheral damage which I could run through. That I did, and finished. The next time I tackled 100 miles, I had a full blister-repair kit including scalpel, bandages and tape.

It takes a number of ultra-running events before you crack the pain puzzle. Feel it; decide the cause; do something to alleviate the cause; and then carry on despite the pain. At my first multi-day ultra, I was so naive that I didn't know there was a puzzle to solve.

I entered my first multi-day ultra as preparation for tackling the MDS, so that I could learn what ultra-running in challenging terrain on multiple days is all about. This was a two-day 66 mile race along the North Downs Way in southern England, with an overnight stop in school buildings at the half-way point. Participants could enjoy a hot shower, warm food and a place to park their sleeping bag on the gymnasium floor. It had none of the deprivations of the MDS, but was still tough. At registration, you could drop off a bag with your sleeping bag and change of clothes to be transported to the overnight stop, so we were running light, without the heavy packs required to cross the Sahara. The distance each day was longer than I had ever raced before. I thought this might be a relatively easy introduction to multi-day ultra-running; how wrong I was. It was a painful experience because I was stupid. I chose what I thought would be the perfect running shoes. These were a good pair of trail-running shoes which were well worn-in and fitted like a glove (they actually fitted *too* well). I had used these in shorter events and found them to be great. On Day One, there was a slight rub where the shoes were a bit too snug and my shoelaces a bit too tight. Nothing of significance, I thought. That evening, there was blood on my socks and my foot was sore. This is a common outcome of running an ultramarathon and would soon heal given a day or two of rest. The trouble with multi-day ultra-running, as I discovered, is that there is no 'day or two of rest'. Although I had packed fresh socks, I had not packed an alternative pair of shoes. So, Day 2 involved running in that same pair of trail shoes, with the same snug fit, and the legacy of the first day's rubbing. The situation got worse quickly on Day 2 and I completed the day in pain, with blood seeping through the socks and visible on the outside of the shoe uppers. So, I endured the pain, and I finished, but it was so unnecessary and not enjoyable. My first thought was, if this is multi-day ultra-running, you can keep it.

I learned several lessons from my first ultra-distance running event. First, buy trail-running shoes at least half a size bigger than you are used to, perhaps a full size larger. Second, wear two pairs of socks, testing out combinations until you find the combination that works for you. Third, if there is the slightest niggle or uncomfortable rub, accept the loss of time to stop, take off your shoes and deal with the cause. This does not make you immune to blisters, but it *does* give your body the best chance to delay the onset of painful damage. Once the skin is broken, there is no let-up until the race is over. For the MDS, this is a full week later. Whilst in the desert, I had never seen such dreadfully damaged feet amongst the MDS participants. For my part, I had learnt my lesson. This earned me a few days relatively pain free in the first half of the week before the inevitable damage of sustained desert running took its toll.

This chapter is mostly about accepting and embracing pain as the inevitable consequence of ultra-running. That is not always the best advice. Sharp localized pain indicates that there is an injury requiring attention. In training, I advocate that you always back off, and if it endures, stop. The rule-of-thumb for me is that any specific pain, even quite small, requires three days of rest. Don't worry about your training plan being scrapped; instead, learn to enjoy the pleasure of not training. True, the pleasure of not training is something people of my age tend to over indulge. But it *is* fun not to train, provided it is a temporary respite that does not degenerate into sloth. When you train regularly, taking time out should be seen as a pleasure to be enjoyed. There is a negative mindset that can get hold of zealous ultra-runners, that they must continue to run, come what may. As you get older, your body is less able to repair itself, and slower to recover, so should be given time. Continuing to run while ignoring injury risks turning minor damage into a severe, chronic long-term problem. Enjoy the break, and when you do resume, start easy.

When the self-medication of three days' rest does not fix it, you may need medical advice. There have been times when doctors have queried why I am still running at my age. I would not go back to any doctor who said that to me, and if any health practitioner suggests that you are too old to run, you need to find a new one. No older person should accept such dismissive attitudes. I can understand the medical profession's frustration with people of my age who are lazy and overweight and yet expect a magic pill to restore their health. Those of us in our seventh decade or beyond, who still strive to maintain an active life, should continue to have full access to medical support. After all, remaining active is the best medicine you can take. There are of course excellent doctors and nurses, and their advice can be reassuring. Years after returning from the Sahara, I did finally have a go at an even tougher race, the UTMB. Ten days before an important qualifying race, I got injured. For my final days of training, I had gone running in the Black Mountains in South Wales. I was running wearing the clothes I would be wearing in the race, consisting of shorts and long pressure socks. The weather had been hot and I had rolled down the socks. The extra pressure around my ankles had caused the sheath around my Achilles tendon to rub and then inflame. After completing the mountain training session, I drove home, arriving to find that my ankle had swelled badly. The race was only ten days away and my attendance was in jeopardy.

My doctor was understanding, having come to know how much ultra-running means to me. I was referred immediately to a physiotherapist, who was also sympathetic. He examined my swollen ankle and concluded that despite appearances, there was minor damage to the Achilles tendon sheath rather than anything major. He carried out a massage to move some of the fluid, gave me a set of gentle exercises and stretches to do, and booked a further appointment a few days hence. At the second appointment, it was still painful but the swelling was less. It was now only a week before the 100 km mountain race in the Alps. I wanted the physio's advice as to whether I could run. I admit to taking quite an aggressive approach of indicating that it was my intention to run unless told not to. His verdict was that I would likely do no lasting damage if I raced through the pain, with the caveat to stop if it got significantly worse. That was the advice I wanted to hear; I had the green light to do the race.

The race was fine. It was brutal and I had been completely wiped out, nothing unusual there. The pain around my Achilles tendon had been my constant companion but it hadn't escalated, so I had ignored it through to the finish. I could do that only by leaning on medical advice. If pain had started during the race, indicating injury, running through it would not have been sensible. When you are within the mental compartment of an ultra race, not succumbing to pain is essential if you are going to finish. That does not mean you suspend logic. Some types of pain arise from fatigue and soreness that can be ignored, but you need to recognize when the discomfort indicates an injury that requires that you stop.

Pain and ultra-running are bedfellows. To take up ultra-running in order to experience the pain would be exceedingly odd, in my view, but pain is an integral part of the ultra-runner's lot. If you regard pain as something to avoid, ultra-running is probably not for you. If you were to persevere and enter the strange and special world of ultra-running, you could get caught in the trap of popping painkillers. If pain puts you off to this extent, I suggest that you try another, less extreme activity. It is not for me to say what that might be. Playing golf or setting out on easy country walks might be a better choice. Better to do that than become reliant on medication.

I suggest there are good reasons to take up ultra-running. Do it for the challenge; for the extreme emotions it engenders; for the sheer joy of moving through rugged remote terrain; and for the satisfaction of learning how to compartmentalise and deal with pain. Enjoy the running; enjoy the challenge; enjoy the pain.

CHAPTER 4

ULTRA-RUNNING AS MEDICINE

Doctors don't prescribe ultra-running.

Your doctor will encourage you to take regular exercise, such as a daily walk. Owning a dog might help to make this a habit by giving you a duty to walk the dog. Exercise classes are also a good way to get a greater variety of movement and to utilize a wider range of muscles. Pilates is one choice for low-impact gentle exercise. For more intense exercise, you could explore a branded exercise class such as Zumba or get involved in indoor cycling by joining a spin class. It is widely accepted by health professionals that persuading older people to be active ensures that they are physically independent for as long as possible. It is good for the pensioners involved and saves money by delaying the need for medical intervention.

Yet while doctors will encourage physical activity for pensioners, they don't generally recommend ultra-running because it carries appreciable risks. It is much safer to advise patients to refrain from strenuous physical exercise and let the normal course of ageing take its toll. Short bursts of hard strenuous exercise, where there is a risk of rupturing something, is indeed suitable and safe only for younger people. The physical stress of ultra-running can be extreme but the cardiovascular stress is low, so it has no age limit. Despite the knowledge that ultra-running for older people is likely to extend the period of active good health, it is a brave doctor who advises patients to take up this slow-burn version of extreme physical exercise. It has the potential to slow the physical degradation of ageing, allowing the patient to remain fit and healthy until their final run. If a patient dies whilst out running, it might be assumed that running was the cause. It is safer, professionally, for doctors to provide risk-adverse medical advice that goes no further than recommending gentle exercise. This should insulate the doctor from bereaved relatives looking for reasons to hold the doctor to account. It is a shame that what may be best for the patient might be obscured by this culpability game.

Like much of effective healthcare, patients should take more responsibility for their own health. I have chosen to take up ultra-running as I get older in order to avoid a long period of poor mobility and ill health, accepting the risk that my final breath might be taken whilst out running. Only you, the patient, can decide that being a regular runner will provide you with a healthier outcome. The risk that running could finish off an old person is, in my view, a risk outweighed by the potential improvement in their quality of life. This is not formal medical advice; it is simple common sense. It is easier for the patient to decide this, though, than for the doctor.

Medical knowledge and capabilities have never been better. We should be the healthiest generation there has ever been. Why is it, then, that many older people enter a downward spiral of failing health? Why is it that society shoulders the costs of an older generation who are increasingly unwell but living longer? I suggest that is not the fault of medicine nor doctors, but rather the result of choices made by many people as they enter retirement, and a society that accepts slothful behaviour as normal. The term 'retire' implies inactivity; and there is no drug or medical intervention to counter the damage it causes. Retirement from paid work should not be seen as an excuse to do nothing but instead as an opportunity to use the freedom to ramp up physical activity.

Modern medicine has banished many diseases which were once the scourge of humankind. There are now vaccines, antibiotics and drugs for just about every condition. Where potential health problems have a genetic basis, there is even the prospect of gene editing to eliminate the risk. If an organ fails, it can be replaced with one transplanted from a donor. If a joint fails, it can be replaced with an artificial one. There is a long list of medications and procedures to help people live longer, but what is the point if these extra years are lived in poor health?

Using medicine to alleviate symptoms and fix problems when they become manifest is not a healthcare system, but a sickness-management system. With tight medical budgets, resources for programmes that champion healthy lifestyle are limited. This is despite evidence that prevention is better than cure – and should be cheaper in the long run. Entry to the current medical system becomes available once we are ill. The sickness-management system can then provide drugs to alleviate the symptoms or replace joints weakened by sustained inactivity. When you reflect and think, it seems clear that retiring into inactivity turbocharges the ageing process. It is like deciding that the race of life is run, and it is time to sit on the sidelines waiting for the end. It has become accepted that old age in rich developed countries can go on for decades with a daily set of pills and replacement joints as required. We should not accept such slow decline and push instead for continuing to live life full-on until finally the lights go out.

I have pointed the finger of the cause of an epidemic of ill health towards systemic failure. To drive home the point, the system I am criticizing is the whole overall system. Doctors are highly capable, hospitals efficient and drugs generally do what is claimed on the label; the weak part of the system is patient failure to comply with healthy living advice. We live in a free society where people live their lives how they choose, particularly in retirement when the formal demands are few. There is no amount of medical budget that can overcome such patient apathy. Withdrawing or delaying treatment for those who are unwilling to help themselves, or compulsory exercise classes, are possible ways forward but in a democratic free society, the scope for such authoritarian measures is limited. Each of us is free to make healthy lifestyle choices that should mean that our personal medical support system works. And yet it doesn't. It's poorly resourced because resources go overwhelmingly to the those who have inflicted ill health on themselves. Although the National Health Service in the UK is overstretched, my personal experience is that when I turn up without the obvious signs of self-neglect, doctors have given me a good hearing. If I were a doctor – which the reader should remember I am not – I would rather give my time to people who live a healthy life but are dealt the card of illness rather than manage the ill health of those whose lifestyle makes it inevitable.

Entering the final stage of life, hoping for a long life, is of little use unless we are well enough to enjoy it. The potential benefits of modern medicine are being squandered by relying too much on it. Living our lives expecting doctors to have a prescription or procedure to fix any health problem is a fool's paradise. The body is exceedingly good at doing its best to stay healthy – given the opportunity. Medical intervention should be reserved for relatively rare occasions, such as an attack by a virus or other pathogen, an accident or the unpredictable lottery of cancer. Medicine does not have the cure for self-inflicted neglect brought on by lack of physical activity, perhaps amplified by a poor diet. Rather than lean on medicine, good health should be promoted through activity such as ultra-running. Running regularly and slowly uses the joints, keeping them healthy, and gently jolts the skeleton, keeping the bones strong.

If you go through middle age with a lazy attitude to exercise, you will enter the inevitable decline of old age with a flying start. That was me aged fifty-eight. I had been a triathlete in my younger days, but a severe road traffic accident in my late thirties had brought my racing days to an abrupt end. Whilst out training on my bicycle, I was hit head-on by a car travelling at speed. My recollections of the incident are limited to the moment before impact and then waking in hospital. A long period of rehabilitation followed, during which it was suggested that my running days were over. The main medical intervention through the period of rehabilitation were the physiotherapists, who got me to do deceptively gentle and easy exercise routines. My recovery was frustratingly slow but over a period of months the regular exercise worked its magic, forcing my body to fix itself. This was clear evidence to me of physical activity as medicine. After about eighteen months, I could handle short-duration runs and was relieved to be able to live a normal active life. As my focus switched to family and career, I did not try to return to racing.

Through my forties and fifties, I felt well enough, was not noticeably overweight and, overall, a normal healthy middle-aged man. It was only when I decided to mark my sixtieth birthday by doing something special that I discovered the truth. Building up my strength to be able to compete in the MDS exposed how weak and unfit I had become. Physical decline had crept up on me. I suppose I allowed myself the conceit of believing I was still an athletic person even though it was no longer true. When I look around at people my age, I see that such self-deception is widespread. I could accept being normal compared with others in modern society, and enter the path laid out of failing health and reduced mobility – or I could do something different.

There is a tendency for medical issues to be a focus of discussion in social conversation amongst older people. This is not surprising because there may be little else of significance going on in their lives. I would rather such discussions remained within my close family, so tend not to join in. In writing I do not wish to dwell on my own health but unless I touch on my medical circumstances, you, the reader, might be left with the wrong impression. It may seem that my late conversion to ultra-running has worked for me because I have been lucky to have been dealt a good set of genes which can handle the punishment. Perhaps ultra-running is not for every old person but for a few particularly resilient and healthy people. That is not true, and by sharing some of my own medical history I can demonstrate that.

A while after completing the MDS, I was invited to participate in a heart-health study of endurance athletes. I was flattered to be referred to as an 'endurance athlete' and happy to be involved. I felt good, fit and well. I had not had a reason to see a doctor for many years and was not on any medication. If my involvement would help the research that would be great; and there could be no harm in a free MOT. I signed a form to allow my data to be used in the research, with the small print stating that if anything was picked up, I agreed that it could be shared with my doctor. I was looking forward to showing just how fit and well an ultra-runner in their sixties can be. I reported to a hospital in London on a Sunday when the researchers had access to equipment fully utilized for treating patients during the working week. I was put on an exercise bike whilst wired up with electrodes stuck all over my torso and I ramped up the power until I ran out of puff. We were then placed in an MRI scanner to take detailed picture of heart and surrounding arteries. The watts I could push out on the bike and my low resting pulse rate all indicated I was in tip-top shape.

I received a letter, a few weeks later, thanking me for my involvement. The letter was copied to my doctor as it advised that I should be referred to a cardiovascular consultant, without explaining why. I was surprised and a little concerned. I supposed that the researchers had a duty of care to be double safe and hoped that it would be nothing serious. My doctor put me on statins and low-dose aspirin as a precaution and referred me to the cardiologist at my local hospital. When I had the initial appointment, the consultant cardiologist listened to my heart, took my blood pressure and pulse and said all appeared to be fine and that I seemed very fit and well. He also said he could see no need for the statins or aspirin. However, just to be sure, he would arrange for the researchers to pass my heart scans to him. I felt reassured and relieved, as it had been preying on my mind that there might be something wrong. The second appointment with the cardiologist was a different matter. He had examined the scans and was surprised I had showed no symptoms. The words in his report were that I had 'severe burden of calcified coronary atheroma'.

I have reluctantly accepted that severe calcification of my arteries, once you have it, does not go away. I need to take a cocktail of drugs for the rest of my life. This is despite no symptoms, and I still participate in ultramarathons. I assume that my blocked arteries are the legacy of a lazy middle age. If I had not got hooked on ultra-running and then volunteered for research, the first indication might have been a heart attack. I believe that ultra-running has saved me. Promoting ultra-running is not taught in medical schools as a way to manage severe coronary blockages. I can see why. Prescribing cholesterol-lowering drugs can improve the blood test numbers so that when I die (as we all do), my medical notes can show that the doctors did their best. If they prescribed ultra-running, when I die, which would likely to be whilst out running, they will be blamed. Only you, the patient, can make the brave decision say: sod it, I am going to run until the lights go out.

The medical facts about getting old are well understood, but we leave dealing with them until it is too late. This is unfortunate, as there are effective measures to manage this life transition. First, prevention is better than cure. Second, consider lifestyle change before drugs. Third, ramping up physical activity is better than winding down. Doctors are well placed to reinforce this message with advice to healthy older people, but they don't have the time, and few people can afford a private physician to offer such advice. All too often, we book an appointment with the doctor only when symptoms are apparent and then demand that the doctor provides a drug to cure us. In the UK National Health Service, where appointments are typically ten minutes, there is no time to extol the virtues of healthy living. This means you must take charge of your own health. This is particularly important in old age as the body weakens and the potential for ill health increases. Yes, of course, go to the doctor, but without symptoms, you will be sent packing as a time-waster. You need to start, before you have symptoms, to fix it yourself: to prevent ill health, improve lifestyle and get active.

The twin objectives of the medical support provided to older people are to prolong life and improve its quality – but the sequencing is usually wrong. Prolonging life tends to attract the most attention and most medical resources, but I argue that it should be the second priority. The priority should be to feel fit and well for as long as possible. A period of failing health leading to death is to be expected, but presumably not much fun. Some people spend decades slowing down, doing less, feeling ill, needing personal care, and perhaps finally confined to bed. Instead of maintaining a good standard of independent personal mobility, older people may go through a transition from using a stick to support walking to dropping down to a shuffle using a Zimmer frame, progressing to riding a mobility scooter, and finally being wheeled around in a wheelchair. Of course, use a stick if you need it, but the latter stages of this progressive loss of independence and mobility must be soul-destroying. It is also resource intensive, and unfair on relatives forced to become carers. The gold standard of a good death is to be fit and well until the day you die. You can stack the odds in your favour of achieving this by the choices you make in retirement.

I do not advocate driving your body hard to stay super fit, because of the risk that it might break down under the intense pressure. This is fine for young athletes but not for old codgers like me. It may work in ensuring you feel good but the time you have left might be curtailed. A balanced approach is required to deliver an extended old age of high-quality living. Each person will age in their own way, so a universal approach to how to slow its progress and remain well until the end is not possible. This book is about using ultra-running to achieve this end, but it may not suit everyone.

There is an important lesson here. Longevity and quality of life are different issues. I want high quality of life until the very end. By continuing to ultra run into old age, I expect to remain feeling fit, until one day I keel over dead. I hope that is not any time soon, but I have no intention of backing off and as a result descending into many years of failing health, popping pills, getting slower and less mobile. The medical community is great when you need it, but self-help should come first. Get outside, get active, get running.

CHAPTER 5

BODY MAINTENANCE

The worst damage you can do to your body
is not to use it.

Running requires every part of your body to work together in concert: muscles to provide power; skeleton to carry the load; and ligaments to hold it all altogether. These need to be in tip-top shape, and the routine of ultra-running can ensure they are. The modest stress of ultra-running is ideal for building a resilient body and strong cardiovascular system, delaying the process of physical ageing. There are particular parts of the body which need to be looked after carefully in order to ultra-run with confidence. These are the feet, knees and bum.

Feet

The general guidance for looking after feet is to be very protective. Any damage, no matter how small, will escalate during the course of an ultra-distance event, particularly if it takes place over a number of days. The most obvious issue is what you wear on your feet, but the first lesson is to prepare them well. An odd tip I was given is that tanned feet have stronger skin. I have no idea if this is true, but sitting outside in the sun with bare feet, allowing the sun to get to them, is an enjoyable training session. Another piece of advice that I know to be true is to cut your toenails. In one 100 mile race, I lost both big toenails; it wasn't pleasant. I now cut them as short as possible, improving the chances that they will remain attached to my feet.

Having taken measures to achieve leathery feet and short toenails, these need to be protected by running shoes. There has been a fad for minimalist running shoes that allow the feet freedom to run almost as if they were bare. These might work for top athletes and fast light runners, but not for elderly plodders. We need comfort and cushioning to be able to run slowly for many hours. There is no magic formula for selecting running shoes, except to try out a range of models until you find a pair that works for you. Shoes need to have space to prevent rubbing, so choose a size which is half or a full size larger than for normal running. The danger here is that feet can move about in the excessive space, thus negating the benefits. This is where your running style can help protect your feet. The idea is to run smoothly, landing without a sheering force between foot and shoe. It would be ridiculous to ask fast runners to do this as they need to drive the pace. In the world of slow running, minimizing the drive you exert saves energy, and saves your feet. A crucial part of your foot protection plan, therefore, is to wear two pairs of socks. I like to wear a pair of toe socks closest to my foot. These are made of thin cotton material that covers each toe individually, ensuring no rubbing of toe on toe. On top of this, I wear a second pair of normal socks. Where there is movement between the foot and the shoe, the rubbing is between one sock and the other, thus protecting the skin on the feet.

For trail running, it is important that the soles have good grip and strong uppers to protect the feet. A toe box is useful as it is impossible to avoid rock-kicking when running over rough terrain, as I discovered in the Sahara. I came across a long, flat stretch of empty and featureless desert littered liberally with black rocks each no larger than 10cm across. Had I not been so tired, I might have bounded over these small obstacles. Doing the ultra-run shuffle, though – despite focussing hard – it proved impossible not to kick a rock every few hundred metres. The first kick is annoying as your toes hit the inside front of the shoe; the second more so; the tenth hurts; and many more hits end up drawing blood.

The Sahara had further foot-related challenges. The prospect of racing for a week through the desert was fearsome in many respects; worrying about my feet was just a relatively minor concern. I fretted about the heat, the sun and the energy-sapping soft sand. I had read reports of sand getting into running shoes and cutting feet to ribbons, having a similar effect to wearing sandpaper instead of socks. After a lot of reading, experimentation and testing, I homed in on what proved to be a winning combination.

The key to healthy feet in the desert is keeping out the sand. The solution is sand gaiters. I bought and tested a couple of models and much depended on how well they attached to the shoes. The gaiters I selected required Velcro to be glued securely around the perimeter of the shoe just above the sole. Before fitting this, I decided on the pair of shoes I wanted to use in the race. I ran in them a few times to confirm my choice. I then purchased an identical pair. One pair was fitted with Velcro and put aside for the race. The other pair I used for training.

There was one final test. I took the race shoes and gaiters to the sand dunes at Perranporth on the Cornish coast in southwest England. I ran for 5 km over soft sand dunes, which was knackering. That test gave me an indication of just how brutal the MDS was going to be, and it did make me think twice about whether I was up to the challenge. In the desert, I was to encounter taller dunes than those at Perranporth and which extended over much longer distances. The double-marathon stage had one stretch of high dunes of soft sand that continued without respite for over 20 km. By then, I was into the event and no way out except through. In the Perranporth dune test, the Velcro came adrift from the shoe. The glue was strong, but clearly not strong enough. Further research discovered that it is common for the Velcro to come adrift during the pounding of the MDS. Repair would be difficult in the desert. Therefore, in addition to gluing, I sewed the Velcro to the shoe with extra-strong thread. I was so glad I did: many people had their feet trashed by the ingress of sand. The gaiters I wore came back from the Sahara tattered and damaged, with no more mileage left in them, but they had done the job required of them.

Knees: use them or lose them

The worst damage you can do to your knees is not to use them. Without regular stress, the ligaments and supporting muscles weaken with old age. The weakness will not be obvious from one day to the next – until that is, you slip or trip, and your knee cannot handle the unexpected load. The resulting injury might be used as a further excuse to use the knees even less. Doctors may be of little help prescribing painkillers to mask the symptoms. Uninterrupted, this cycle of decline may lead eventually to knee replacement. The cause is not overuse, but underuse. Breaking the cycle means ramping up exercise in a steady progression towards stronger knees. To all those older people who repeat the mantra, 'I no longer run to protect my knees', my response is 'hogwash'.

The knee joint connects the upper and lower legs and allows it to articulate. For runners, good knee function is key to the running movement. For everyone, knee health is vital to moving around and living life to the full. Knee problems can be a huge damper on quality of life. Ultra-running can be the best medicine to keep your knees healthy and strong into old age, without needing to go under the orthopaedic surgeon's knife.

The bones above and below the knee (femur and tibia) are butted together, held in place by ligaments and tendons connecting the muscle, with cartilage protecting the moving surfaces. It is a very complex joint that is susceptible to injury, if it is not cared for. When little used and not stressed on a regular basis, these components lose their strength. If you don't enjoy strenuous activity, this may not be of concern to you, but it should be. If you have weak knees and allow weakness to continue, then the odd trip or fall might cause damage; the occasional run may also overstress the components and cause damage or injury. So, the occasional run for an overweight inactive older person can indeed be bad for the knees. The particular circumstances of someone who has neglected strength and fitness is not a fair test of whether running is good for the knees. The logical deduction, when the facts are examined, is that neglecting strength and fitness over extended periods is the underlying cause of an epidemic of knee problems in older people. The true solution is to use your knees on a regular basis, using activity such as ultra-running to build strength and protect your knees.

'I don't expect my knees to allow me to continue running when I reach your age,' said a veteran runner twenty years my junior to me at the finish of the Snowdon UTMB race in Wales. On this occasion, I had entered the relatively short 50 km race, which made good use of the distance by going over Mount Snowdon, not just once but twice. It was a hard day out and a hard day for my knees. I was surprised at his comment, and the implication that I was lucky to still be running at my age. His words were intended well but such comments get me riled. It is not that I am lucky; it is because I remain active. Over the years that I've been ultra-running I have heard so many people say to me that they no longer run because of their knees. When I ask why, it might be because their knees hurt when they run, or because they want to protect their knees, or simply an excuse not to bother to get outside and run. These reasons do not add up. I accept that if through sustained low levels of activity, knees have become weak and subsequently damaged, there may be no way back, and in the end a replacement joint is the only solution. It would be so much better to intercept this process of knee decline in the early stages to reverse the direction of travel, building strength and resilience, to keep your knees functioning well into old age.

Ultra-running doesn't insulate you from knee damage, but it does make you much more resilient against injury. The pressure exerted on the knees during ultra-running can be extreme, for example running downhill in the mountains over rocky terrain, especially at night when vision is impaired. Each foot landing could be a slip, or a trip or a fall. One viewpoint is that only those with strong knees will survive such punishment. The reverse view is that the way to get strong knees is to inflict such punishment. What came first, the strong knees or the ultra-running? Is it strong knees that allow you to ultra-run; or ultra-running that strengthens your knees?

Of course, injury is always a possibility that should be guarded against. Not by avoiding the punishment of running, though, but by being careful. Strength training, such as weightlifting and box jumps in the gym, helps, but is not a guarantee of protection. I was injured whilst doing hill intervals near where I live. I don't have mountains close by, but I have found a steep piece of rough terrain. I was putting myself through my paces, striding to the top, running down, time and time again. And again. Stupidly I had worn a pair of old running shoes without much bounce left in them. I was also testing how fast as I could run down hill on such rough ground and stay upright. I didn't notice the rabbit hole hiding in the grass and my right knee caught it. The combination of twisting and high impact did not go well. It was painful to walk for the next few days. I took my standard medicine of three days of rest and then resumed running gingerly. I could have used this as an excuse to finally stop running. If I had, I feel sure I would now be crocked. I backed off for a while, but kept my resolve and then resumed running.

There is no doubt that I had been injured. I didn't go to the doctor, so I do not know what the injury was. The body's repair mechanisms kicked in, guided by my action to continue running at low intensity. This told my body, ever so gently, that I wanted to build it back stronger than before. If I was to sit around doing nothing, especially now that the ageing mechanisms have been activated, my body might not work so hard at making a repair. Whilst writing this paragraph, I wondered how my words might be received. I therefore spoke with a physiotherapist to seek an expert opinion on my non-expert analysis. He explained that the treatment he provides is all about recommending exercises that will speed up and aid recovery. He went onto to explain that his main gripe with his work is people who can't be bothered to do the exercises and still want him to fix them with something easier, such as a pill to swallow. I was castigated for not going to see a physiotherapist to get a professional diagnosis, but the physio agreed entirely that appropriate exercise is the best medicine. Going further, he expressed the view that pills and surgery have little chance of providing the cure unless the patient actively engages in forcing recovery. So, there we have a slam-dunk. Running is good for the knees provided you do it often enough and long enough. That is ultra-running in a nutshell.

During an ultra-running race, your knees can fail you. This is where walking/running poles can help. I used to think that these were for softies. Certainly, walking the streets or flat paths, walking poles are only for those at risk of falling over – and for such people, they are very useful. For those of us with good mobility, poles can be useful to share the load on long, steep mountain ascents. Instead of the thigh muscles doing all the work, the arms can make a contribution. Poles also have other uses.

The 100 km CCC is described by the race organizers as the 'little sister of the UTMB'. It starts in Courmayeur, Italy, traverses through Champex, Switzerland, and ends in Chamonix, France. Entering this race was another step beyond my comfort zone, and a further test of what might be possible. I approached the race with some trepidation, so started to research what it would entail and seek advice. I discovered a briefing day convened by a UK-based race organization to explain the event, what it required of runners and advice on how to prepare. I listened with fascination as Tom Evans, the previous year's winner, gave his account of how he had got ready for the race. Some weeks prior to it, he had gone with a group of friends to walk the route over three days, making notes whilst having a very relaxed and convivial hike with his mates. He explained how he had identified a long, easy incline in the second half of the route that was on a track and easily runnable. He recognized this as his opportunity to win the race by planning to run hard up this long climb at a point in the race when fatigue kicks in. This was an insight into how race winners think and plan – and yet not relevant to me. What was relevant were his views on walking/running poles.

I was sitting in the audience as a pole refusenik. In my ignorance, I had watched other runners at my moderate pace using poles in races and had looked down on them, seeing the poles as a sign of weakness. I had not realized that the fast runners out front and out of my sight were also using poles. My flawed thinking was that running poles were an unnecessary appendage and not worth the bother. As I listened to the previous year's race winner speaking, he advised strongly that we carry poles and use them on the steep sections. His was a voice I respected, so I was persuaded to give them a try. After researching the different options, I bought a pair and started to use them. Out on runs close to home, I felt self-conscious, not wanting to look like people who follow the Nordic walking craze. I was still not convinced that they were particularly useful but I persevered slowly, learning when they were helpful and where they should be folded up and packed away. Eventually, I started to get it. I found that they helped me survive a few big races, where I was exceedingly glad of them. The main surprise for me was to discover that poles really came into play on steep descents. Towards the latter stages of mountain races, my legs would often turn to jelly. It was tiring to descend steep slopes, but it was worse than that; I was struggling even to stay upright. The poles provided the additional stability my wobbly knees required. I am now a strong pole advocate and would not tackle a mountain ultra race without a pair.

Unmentionables

Let us consider the third key body component to look after carefully: the bum. There is nothing more annoying when running blister free, and injury free, than getting a sore bottom. This is particularly painful in hot conditions when salty sweat adds a sting to the discomfort. Generally, this is not a problem over shorter runs, and even up to marathons. Over ultra distances, however, the very slight rubbing of cheek on cheek can cause this most sensitive area to become red raw. The rubbing is almost imperceptible but once the skin is broken, each stride is painful. I have tried to adopt a gait with the legs swinging wider than normal; it doesn't work. Once you have a sore bum, the only way to relieve it is a big dollop of Vaseline between the cheeks. You only experience this particular issue once, as it leaves a distinct and lasting impression. You then add a task to your standard pre-race routine. Smear a finger liberally with Vaseline and reach down the back of the shorts to apply it. You'll need to top up about every 50 km. Do this diligently and sore bum can be eliminated as a source of discomfort.

Finally, having descended into discussion about unmentionable aspects of ultra-running, the need to stop to defecate comes high on the list. Running events will usually provide temporary toilets facilities. These may not be pleasant but are hygienic, provided you remember to take your own toilet paper. On the downside, if you want to evacuate your bowels whilst waiting at the start there is likely to be a long queue. Stopping to use pre-positioned mobile toilets along the route shouldn't delay you much, particularly later in the race when the field is strung out. The issue during the race is that such facilities will be few and far between. Races in mountainous or remote locations may have none at all along the route. More often than not, the urge to dash to the toilet does not coincide with the location of a convenient mobile toilet. That is where you need to find the proverbial bush to squat down behind.

Taking a comfort break in the Desert was particularly challenging. Not surprisingly, there was a distinct lack of bushes. When you are part of a long line of runners crossing featureless terrain, there is nowhere to hide. The standard procedure required dispensing with any qualms you might have and peeling off to the side. In full view of the other runners, you turn back to face your fellow runners, drop your shorts and squat down. The open desert gets a full view but the other runners just meet your gaze, returning a smile of schadenfreude. Where the result is solid, the procedure required by the race organizers was to bag it (in brown plastic bags provided for the purpose) and carry it to the next aid station. With my military background, I did not have a difficulty with such alfresco toileting, but some runners found it embarrassing. This led to one incident of culturally insensitive behaviour.

Every now and then, the race would pass by small communities of just one or two buildings clustered around a water well. These were simple mud huts where local people and their families scratched out a living. They may have been poor and their circumstances hard, but they were proud people, and these buildings were kept neat and orderly. As we passed one such small community, you could see the children playing outside and their mother outside the front of her house watching the spectacle of the race. Then it happened. I don't know what was going through this runner's head, except that she needed to relieve herself. She ran off behind the building to do just that but then reappeared to join the line of runners, being pursued by an extremely angry woman. Believing it would be acceptable to use the vicinity of the local lady's family home as a toilet showed an astounding degree of cultural ignorance. When you run or race, you will have to jettison biodegradable personal waste at some point, but this needs to be somewhere off the path; do it out of sight if you can, and definitely not is someone's backyard.

More could be written about cuts, bruises, blood in urine, and other bodily functions including, heart arrythmia brought on by extreme exertion, but I have written quite enough. In a book that extols the benefits and fun of ultra-running, I have probably written too much already. There is one of the body's organs not mentioned here: the brain. The brain, or rather the mind that resides within it, determines whether you can engage successfully with ultra-running. The importance of that is the subject of the next chapter.

CHAPTER 6

IT'S IN THE MIND

If you believe you can, you can.

Belief is the bedrock of the human mind, guiding decisions, building confidence and providing resilience to whatever life might throw at us. If the mind is fully engaged, the physical body can do extraordinary things. The primacy of the mind is particularly strong in ultra-running. If you believe you can run ultra-marathons, you can. The converse is also true: if you believe you can't, you are unlikely to finish. Ultra-running requires strength of mind, and it helps to develop such strength, with the side-effect of improving overall mental resilience.

When I was younger, ultra-running did not enter my mind as something I might want to do. I saw it at that time as an odd activity carried out by slightly strange people. I assumed anyone could do it, provided they could tolerate the tedium of endless miles. For someone who enjoyed racing, this seemed to be a dull pursuit and not for me. As I got older, with indications that my physical ability was declining, my perception changed. My mind became fascinated by ultra-running as a new challenge. I cannot pretend to understand the minds of other ultra-runners, and I am certainly not a psychiatrist, so what I write here should be treated with caution.

My early forays into ultra-running showed that it is indeed all in the mind. I have been overtaken by people who do not have the look or shape of athletes. I mean no disrespect in writing this; quite the opposite; I found it hugely impressive that they had a mindset which took them over the finishing line – ahead of me.

Initially, I had attempted to run all the way, but couldn't, dropping to a walk for the latter stages. Ambling dejectedly, I was overtaken by people I might have categorized on the start line as 'non-athletic' but who went by running slowly with a metronomic steady pace. I felt that I must be at least as good an athlete as them, but they had something I didn't. This was the mental capability to endure the discomfort and maintain the pace, albeit slowly, when the body is dog tired. This was the background to working out a mental model I could use in subsequent ultra-running races.

Having entered ultra-running at a mature age, I have been able to observe how my mind has adapted to embrace the challenge. The mental model I have adopted supports ultra-running with its strange requirement to keep going when the sensible thing would be to stop. Ultra-running does not do sensible. A state of mind is required which make it possible to run ridiculously long distances, and enjoy it. To achieve this, I separate my mind into two version of me. The first is the 'inner pilot' and the second is the 'emotional self'. These two minds behave differently and interact. Whether they are in harmony (or not), dictates whether I succeed – or not.

My inner pilot is at the core of the mental model. It needs to be strong, in control, and operates using logical analysis. Not so logical perhaps, or the simple logic of protecting self through not ultra-running might take over; but logical enough to make good decisions to safely reach the finish line. The inner pilot makes the decisions and enforces them.

The emotional self, feels, loves, and enjoys or hates what is going on.

Some people may not have developed a dual-mind approach to life. It becomes necessary only when there is a need to deal with extreme situations. I fostered such a mindset whilst serving in the UK airborne forces. This got me through some difficult situations where my emotional self was terrified. Fighting in the 1982 Falklands War was one occasion when my duty and emotions were hugely conflicted and required the steely determination of a strong inner pilot. Prior to this, I had already honed the ability to trick my mind into being cool with parachuting. One incident was amusing and a real eye-opener to the separation between inner pilot and emotional self. We were on a training exercise in southern England which required insertion by parachute at night at low level. I was standing at the open door of the C130 Hercules transport aircraft, staring into the black of the night with the smell of aviation fuel in my nostrils and the roar of the engines in my ears. I was fixated on the red light on the bulkhead. When this switched to green, this was my instruction to jump and lead the long line of troops behind me out into the aircraft slipstream. I looked down at my legs and observed my knees shaking uncontrollably. They wouldn't stop. My emotional self was displaying the physical reactions of sheer terror, but oddly my inner self was totally calm. In airborne forces, not to jump would be to be branded a coward. There was no risk of that; my inner pilot was totally in control. At that moment in time, the two parts of my mind were in totally different places, but both aligned to the same outcome; that is, to jump when the light turned green.

Developing and nurturing my inner pilot has allowed me to appear calm and collected even when my emotional self has been in turmoil. Ultra-running is not terrifying, but the mental agility to deal with terrifying situations is similar to that of the ultra-runner. At its core, the problem is the same; the emotional self is trying to take charge. Let it, and you fall apart, unable to function. In the case of the military, this might be frozen with fear; in ultra-running, unable to continue running. It is normal in an ultra race at somewhere beyond halfway for the emotional self to try to exert control. This is far enough into the race to be completely knackered but not close enough to the finish for the end to be within reach. The emotional self has had enough and wants to wrap it up; the inner pilot keeps driving forward. It is wonderful how when the end is close, within say 5 km of the finish line, the emotional self perks up and carries you through to a euphoric completion.

For an ultra-runner, the inner pilot needs to be dominant to keep the emotional self under control. I assume that anyone can nurture a dual-mind mentality, but as you get older such mental gymnastics may be more difficult to master. For people whose emotional self is dominant, they can no doubt live fulfilling lives, but ultra-running is not for them.

In addition to being able to separate the inner pilot and emotional self, you need to be able to trick your mind into coping with the trials of extreme long-distance running. In developing my mental tactics, I have nurtured three modes of thinking: switched on, switched off and switched channel. In any ultra-race, I would hope to employ all three modes at different stages. Switched on is to be focussed and alert; switched off the opposite. Switched channel is my way to mentally escape from the race completely. These modes of thinking help me to cope with the challenges of ultra-running. This is very personal to me, so not a precise thinking model to copy. This shows how you can play mind games to fool your mind and body to carry on despite extreme tiredness, physical pain and mental anguish.

Switched on could be regarded as normal. In this thinking mode, you are focussed on the race. You are navigating looking carefully for route markers and direction signs. You are aware of time and distance. You might be monitoring performance making mental notes of position and split times. This is therefore the thinking mode that facilitates performing well, but is mentally draining. It works well for shorter races but for ultra-running I find this to be too difficult and too tiring to maintain throughout.

Switched off is much easier. In this method, the mind focuses on staying in the moment without noticing the elapse of time or taking note of position. I used this thinking mode a lot crossing the Sahara. As my first big multi-day race, I simply wanted to complete it. To assist me, I wore a simple watch and did not use the stopwatch function. The watch on my wrist showed the time of day, and that was all. For me, finishing would be to win. It was a whole lot easier to switch off during the toughest stages, living in the moment and suspending the passage of time.

Switched channel is an additional mental mode that I managed to master only after completing a number of ultra races. I had come to realize that I had been racing in beautiful remote locations, such as deserts, the high mountains and the Arctic, without really appreciating them. I remembered aspects of the race, but my recollection of place was hazy. To visit such places and not take in the views, smell the aromas, listen to the sounds and soak up the atmosphere, is to waste the experience. The switched channel thinking mode sets your mind free to leave the race and focus on what is around you. Taking time to enjoy the solitude and beauty of the remote desert. From a trail high in the Alps at night, to look down into the valley at the lights of villages below. To be in the Arctic within a unique ecosystem of strange plants and unusual birds. A hiker might watch, listen, observe and enjoy. An ultra-runner should be able to do the same. In fact, in the latter stages of a long ultra race, participants like me in the middle of the pack, end up hiking for much of the time. We try to run on the flat and downhill but late in the race, with tired legs, the slightest incline becomes a hike. Besides, fast hiking can be quicker than a slow, shuffling run. Switching channel can bring the situation alive in an enjoyable manner, as well as be a distraction from the suffering.

I don't know the mental models that other ultra-runners adopt. Mine is not perfect and has its problems. Switched on is obviously the best for performance and fastest finish time. I feel sure that those who aspire to win are always switched on. That is not for me at my stage in life. I need to enjoy the event, or I simply won't turn up at the start line. Switched off works well for continuing to run despite discomfort and pain but is not good for navigation. I was running a local 50 km race called the 'Hundred Hills'. Without mountains in the vicinity, the race organizers had tried to include as much climbing and descent as they could using the local hills. It was aptly named, going up, down, and over, a hundred or more hills on trails made muddy by rain. I found myself on part of the route where the surface was firmer and a gentle grassy downhill gradient was devoid of trip hazards. I allowed my mind to relax into switched-off mode. I felt good, with my legs striding easily downhill, gravity doing the work. I was woken out of my running stupor by a shout from behind. I had missed a turn, continuing straight on and off the racing route. A fellow runner was calling me back. I retraced a few hundred metres to the turn point, noticing that the sign was large and obvious; you couldn't miss it. I had been too successful at switching off.

My third thinking mode, switch channel, is also not without its dangers. In a micro sense it can be as simple as being distract by the view, tripping and taking a tumble. You would not therefore switch channel when descending on steep and potentially dangerous terrain. There are other potential problems with focussing on enjoying the experience. Competing in an 84 km ultra race in northern Finland, the route followed the Karhunkierros (or 'Bear Trail'). It is an absolute gem of a hiking route for Arctic scenery including following the banks of the Oulanka River. I spent much of the event in switched channel mode, soaking up the sight and sounds of the cascading white water. The race started at 9pm so that we could race through the night, which was not as bad as you might imagine. The race was north of the Arctic Circle in the summer, so it was not fully dark, even at midnight. For most of the Bear Trail there is just one route, so it did not matter whether you followed hiking trail signs or race signs. However, in the central portion of the route – where it is most scenic, and where I was firmly in switched-channel mode – there are alternative route choices to take in certain sights. For this race, I had now purchased a GPS watch. Although I had not mastered how to use it to navigate, it was active to show distance and log my run. At the finish, it showed I had run 4 km more than the race distance. I must have been inattentive to race signs whilst enjoying the interesting terrain and perhaps followed hiking signs. No one had called me back, either because night visibility was poor or because the Finns are a taciturn people who tend not to shout out. For whatever reason, this ultra race had been a bit more ultra than intended, all because I had been in switched-channel thinking mode.

Applying my thinking techniques has helped me to push on when my physical body has had enough. One mental challenge I found difficult to address was the extreme low points. Somewhere beyond halfway, I would be consumed by the feeling of 'why am I doing this?'. I would promise myself to never, ever again get myself into this position. I thought of this as mental weakness, until I started to get honest feedback from other ultra-runners. One of my fellow runners across the Sahara was an experienced ultra-runner, who was always the first to finish each stage out of our small tent group. Over many long evenings in the desert, he admitted that in almost every ultra race he had done, he had gone through a low point of never wanting to enter another one. It was reassuring to hear that I was not alone in having such negative thoughts. Such feelings are common but don't usually survive beyond the euphoria of finishing. You feel so good that you start to erase the negative thoughts that weighed so heavily just a few hours before. After the race, the mind carries out a re-evaluation, usually concluding that the event was a good experience. This might not be immediate, though. This positive spin might take over the memory later the same day, next day, next week, or next month, depending on the degree of painful memories which need to be discarded. For one race – the UTMB – reframing the memory as a positive experience was nigh on impossible.

The UTMB is the pinnacle of ultra-distance mountain trail running, involving 100 miles of steep ascent and descent to circumnavigate Mont Blanc traversing through France, Italy and Switzerland. The race starts and ends in the town of Chamonix in the French Alps. I arrived in Chamonix a couple of days before the race, thinking that I was well prepared and was looking forward to the race.

My captivation with the UTMB had developed over the years following the Sahara race. I had discovered that the statement attributed to the MDS, that it was the 'toughest foot race on the planet', was false. The MDS was tough, but the UTMB is tougher. The thought had still not taken root that I might be able to raise my game and take it on. Like a piece of music trapped in my brain as an ear worm, the idea kept playing but always with the same dissonant final chord that I would be incapable of finishing.

As my fascination with ultra-running increased, I couldn't eliminate entirely the possibility of doing the UTMB. As mentioned in Chapter 5, I was drawn towards testing my ability by entering the 100 km CCC, which is the second half of the UTMB, starting in Courmayeur and finishing in Chamonix. Although only half the UTMB beast, it had all the atmosphere of the big event. That race had been a mental and physical challenge that I was proud to have overcome to finish. It was so tough, mentally and physically, that the experience confirmed that the full UTMB was not for me.

That said, I still could not eliminate the UTMB from my mind. It kept thinking about it, each time dismissing it as impossible. Eventually my curiosity led me to investigate whether I might be eligible to enter. I found that with the results from the 100 km CCC, combined with my result from a 100 mile trail race in the UK, I had built up enough points to enter the main UTMB race. So, I had overcome the hurdle of qualification to enter; no mean feat in itself. That meant there was nothing stopping me, except my continued feeling that the UTMB beast would be beyond what I could handle.

Finally, I capitulated to the allure of the UTMB, and entered, despite my severe apprehension.

Looking back, I can see now there was no avoiding my having a go at this big race. Had I not tried, I would always have regretted it, even though I knew it would be likely to beat me.

I prepared as well as possible, in my view. I searched out the steepest and highest hills close to where I live and ran up and down them for hours at a time. Going further afield, I spent whole days in the Welsh mountains, designing routes that crisscrossed to take in as much climbing and descending as possible. I practised night running along rough trails wearing my trusty old head torch. I became adept at looking down at the pool of light in front of me to avoid the tree roots and other trip hazards. I tested several pairs of shoes and purchased a new ultra-light racing backpack. I had done the training; I had the kit; I was ready to go – or so I thought.

The race start was in the early evening with a rousing send-off and plenty of razzmatazz. The first 8 km or so was on roads and the pace was high. It felt like the start of a 10 km race, as I was sucked along with the pack of runners. I found out why the pace was so fast as we hit the steep slopes of narrow mountain paths. The pack of runners became a long snaking line, and over-taking proved difficult. People had been racing off the start line for a place towards the front of the pack. On the steep mountain paths, the pace slowed to something more manageable as we settled into our collective stride.

As night fell, we were in the high mountains and I turned on my head torch. Ascending was hard work but safe, with each stride a deliberate step onto the next rock. Descending was potentially dangerous as I tried to stay upright, stepping from rock to rock in quick succession as gravity took control. This was tiring, mentally and physically. In hindsight, I should have tested how I would fare by entering more night events before attempting the full UTMB. As it was, it was only when I was within the maelstrom of the UTMB that I discovered that the head torch I was wearing was no match for the lights worn by other runners. Running alone at night on familiar trails near home it had been fine with just enough light to run safely. I had not anticipated what it would be like running as a pack. The head torches of runners behind were like searchlights, so powerful that all I could see in front of me was my own dark shadow with the detail of the ground immediately ahead obliterated. My puny head torch was outshone by the other runners', making it next to useless with regard to placing my next foot landing. On the ascents this didn't matter, as we picked our way relatively slowly up the trail. On the rapid descents, it was lethal. I was focussing hard to see a landing spot for each stride, but I was blind in the one place that really mattered: right in front of me. I suffered several trips and tumbles. Without clear vision, I made several bad choices. How ironic that I was running amongst other runners in a sea of light, but I couldn't see the one thing I needed to see: where my feet would land next. This was mentally draining, disconcerting and felt dangerous. It turned out that the danger was very real, as I will describe when I write more about mountain running in Chapter 10.

After 50 km, I arrived at a checkpoint at about 2am. Fifty km is always a psychological milestone for me. Up to the 42 km point, you can tell yourself it is only a marathon; beyond that, you are enter ultra-running territory. The way I was feeling reminded me that 50 km in the mountains is a lot harder than that 50 km on the flat. This was far enough into the race for my emotional self to be tired and my overall mindset negative. As I grabbed something to eat, I was thinking about the next stage back up into the mountains in the dark. My emotional self was not just tired, but also scared. My inner pilot was trying to get a grip to force me to continue. However, the inner pilot was also thinking through the logic. This next stage in the mountains would be dangerous until the light of dawn returned my vision. That was bad enough, but this was the full UTMB, which would require a second night in the mountains. The promise I had made to my wife to stay safe came back to me. The choice was between leaving the aid station to climb back up into the mountains relying on my inadequate head torch, or quit. Not surprisingly, my emotional self wanted to wrap it in but I found that the logic thinking of my inner pilot was advising the same. I felt quite terrible at exiting this way but my two minds were aligned. I knew that this was the right choice but felt such a failure to have been so poorly prepared and weak in my execution.

I approached the race organizers to declare my intention to drop out of the race. I was asked if I was sure of my decision despite no serious injury or signs of exhaustion – beyond what is normal in ultra racing. It was explained that once I was removed from the race, that would be final. The volunteer I approached suggested that I go to the next aid station and then see how I feel. I felt so bad about dropping out that I could easily have been persuaded, but I was resolute; I had made my decision and stuck by it, knowing that if I was weak in that moment I would be back into the steep mountains at night with a feeble head torch. A more senior member of the race crew asked me directly if I was sure that I wanted to withdraw. I felt far from sure, conflicted between accepting failure and the foolhardiness of continuing, but I replied 'yes'. The timing chip on my race number was cut away and I slunk off into a corner at the back of the mountain hut being used for the aid station. I sat with my head in my hands shaking with emotion. The mental anguish was intense. It was not relief I felt but huge disappointment. I had been defeated. I had failed.

There then came a slow tortuous process of getting back to Chamonix. I put on all my emergency clothing to try to stay warm, as I was no longer generating the heat of running. If I had been injured, or taken ill with a heart attack, I would have been quickly and efficiently evacuated. As a dropout, I was nobody. I was simply a piece of race detritus to be cleared off the course in due course. I felt like a fraud and a failure. I had attempted the full format UTMB, and it had beaten me. This should have confirmed that the big beast of the UTMB was not for me.

This was not to be my last attempt at the UTMB, however. It had me gripped and it would not let go.

CHAPTER 7

FEASTING AND FASTING

To eat when you are truly hungry is culinary nirvana.

With a wide variety of food readily available, people who live in affluent developed countries should be the best-nourished generation in human history. The fact that this is not the case is a poor reflection on people's food choices. Part of the problem is people are distracted by the pleasure of eating. Overindulging beyond what the body needs not only leads to health problems, but also dulls the experience of eating. The taste of food is to be enjoyed, but if the appetite has already been sated, there is little true pleasure from forcing down more. This is where ultra-running can help to maintain and enhance the enjoyment of eating. To eat when you are truly hungry, and your body is craving food, is culinary nirvana.

When considering what to eat whilst ultra-running, there are a range of approaches and it is not always obvious what works best. Experimenting to explore options and listening to your body are better than following guidance in the running magazines. In particular, be wary of so-called energy sport drinks, many of which should be classified as junk food. In sustained slow running, fuel is readily available in the reserves of body fat which can be metabolized for energy. Even the leanest runner has fat reserves to last many days. What your body really needs is the nutrition for repair and recovery such as protein, vitamins and minerals.

When out running alone, I like to eat very little, reaping the benefits of immediate detoxification as your body burns through whatever is in your system. This has the additional psychological benefit of lining up an appetite for a really good feed after the run. This has been my habit for many years, having rebelled against the idea that you need to guzzle energy bars and calorific drinks to run long distances. As a 23-year-old, I embarked on one long hike/run in Tasmania from Cradle Mountain to Lake St Clair, a spectacularly beautiful 80 km through stunning scenery populated by unusual antipodean vegetation. This had been a completely unplanned adventure and, in hindsight, perhaps not sensible. I was hitch-hiking through Tasmania, travelling light, and staying in whatever accommodation I came across. One lift was with a man of Scottish heritage who invited me to have dinner with him and his wife and stay the night. The only payment required was to join him in drinking whisky and talk late into the night about the UK. A small price to pay.

In the morning with a slightly thick head, he suggested I should go and see Cradle Mountain. He offered to drive me there, dropping me off at the tourist car park. He explained that there would be so many tourists passing through that it should be easy for me to get an onward lift from there. Arriving at the Cradle Mountain car park, it was a lovely sunny day in early spring with the peaks in clear view. I walked along a path that was signposted towards Lake St Clair. It had steps and a handrail, looking like an easy hike. Without any fixed agenda to constrain me, I set off, not fully registering just how far it would be. As I walked further from the car park, the well-trodden path forged by day-trippers became an ill-defined walking trail marked in places by poles stuck in the ground. Chatting with hikers coming the other way, wearing gaiters and laden with heavy packs, they explained that the marker poles were to mark the trail when the ground is covered in snow. They further explained, not entirely helpfully, that at this time of year there could still be another heavy dollop of snow, so better to be prepared. It forced me to reflect on my circumstances. It was warm and sunny; visibility was good and the track route initially was easy to discern. The map I carried was a free tourist map covering the whole of Tasmania. The Cradle Mountain to Lake St Clair hiking route was depicted by just a few cm on the paper. The map was shaded to show the elevation but, at such a small scale, only the biggest mountains were highlighted. The unobstructed views and perfect weather allowed me to identify these high peaks to get a general steer of my direction, but otherwise I was dependent on following the track, which – as the hike progressed – was in some places indistinct and difficult to follow. Not expecting to be hiking, I was carrying a small backpack but had no compass, head torch or a sleeping bag. I did have hitchhiking gear, consisting of a wash bag, set of spare clothes, a raincoat, bottle of water and an apple. Prepared for an ultra-run in the mountains I was not. With the wisdom of age, I would not repeat this now, but in the rashness of youth, I didn't appreciate the risks I was taking.

As I hiked – and in places jogged – I came to realize that perhaps I was a little exposed and might be in difficulty if the weather turned. I pressed on until dark, stopping for the night at one of the hiking huts along the route. There was a group of students cooking what smelt like good food. I joined in socially and turned down their offer of sharing some of their food, knowing they would have carried only what they needed. I put on my coat and slept as best I could on the hard boards. As soon as dawn broke, and it was light enough to see, I pressed on up the trail, leaving the other people asleep. I was keen to get to the end whilst the weather was still good. The trail was distinct and well trodden at first, but once I arrived at the top of a steep cliff with great views, it ended. I hunted around but saw no footpath going beyond that point. I had no choice but to retrace a few kms back to the hut. The students were starting to wake up. I asked to see one of their hiking maps. I could then see that the trail I had just walked was an optional off-shoot to take in the scenic view. That was something I didn't need. The main trail set off in a different direction. I memorized the map as best I could and headed off, bidding them farewell. I picked my way through the temperate rain forest, marvelling at how wonderful it was and admiring the spring flowers, but most of all I was focussed on not losing the trail.

I arrived at Lake St Clair early afternoon with some relief at getting away with my rather stupid challenge, as well as a huge appetite. A small hotel was serving a three-course Sunday lunch. I sat at a table outside, so as not to annoy other diners with my grubby appearance, and ordered the three-course set menu. After finishing the dessert, I ordered the set menu again. I ate my way through a further three courses. That would normally be regarded as gluttony, but in the circumstance was pure pleasure. I then took a long siesta, lying on the grass in the sun, before getting on my way and hitching my next lift.

I was reminded of just how much I enjoy eating during the food deprivation of the week-long race across the Sahara. The rules of the MDS are quite specific. The only food you have available is the food you carry. The more you pack, the heavier your backpack. Like many other runners, I carried only the minimum required by the race regulations, including nuts and dried foods.

My food plan for the desert race focussed on nutrition in as dense a form as possible. For breakfast, perhaps unwisely, I designed my own special recipe of dry ingredients. I remember preparing these before flying to Morocco, mixing the ingredients into a paste held together by coconut oil. I divided the resulting brown lump into small dense patties, one for each day. I had covered these in cling film, to be unwrapped each morning. The diet was so restricted during the desert race that I usually looked forward to any chance to eat. Breakfast was the exception. I have no recollection now as to the particular ingredients of these brown balls, but I do remember clearly that they tasted terrible. I had taken my search for dense nutrition too far. There was no pleasurable breakfast in the desert for me; only forcing down another brown lump to fuel my body through another hard day. During the day, the menu was better and included a variety of food bars made of nuts and dried fruit. At the end of each stage, I had a sachet of recovery powder to mix with water, to both hydrate and replenish minerals, vitamins and protein. The food highlight of the day was a freeze-dried meal. Runners wanting the lightest possible pack would eat this cold. I preferred to dine with a bit more enjoyment so carried an ultra-light stove and pot to boil water, so that I could spoon a warm meal out of the sachet.

I needed to plan the menu for the rest day. This came midrace after the longest stage, which had been a double marathon. The distance underplays how difficult it was, as the stage had included an energy-sapping stretch over a series of giant sand dunes. Slower participants needed to run through the night into the rest day to complete this most brutal stage. I finished the long stage in the early hours of the rest day, so I had the entirety of it to chill out. Well not exactly, considering the desert heat. I spent it lounging under the shade of the black hessian shelter. This was open on all sides with views out across the desert, a gentle breeze alleviating the stifling heat. It was pure pleasure to be infused with the atmosphere of the desert, sheltered from the sun, and not required to run.

My logic when planning my rest-day food was that as I would not be running, I would not need much, focussed on keeping my pack ultra-light. To have dined well during the rest day would have meant carrying more through the preceding days and I did not want to inflict that on me. What I did inflict on myself was an exceedingly hungry rest day. All I had was a single bag of mixed nuts. I spent the day in relaxed mode, drinking plenty of water (ample water was provided) and deciding which nut I would eat next. I would pick it out of the bag, roll it in my fingers savouring the moment, before putting it in my mouth and eating it ever so slowly. Back in civilization, such a bag of nuts might be munched down as a quick snack almost without thinking. In the desert, it became the focus of intense sustained pleasure. How one pack of nuts could allow me to dine like a king reminds me how much of the food we eat day-to-day is swallowed with little thought and little true enjoyment.

That rest day in the desert had another pleasant surprise in store. The race was controlled with daily final cut-off times. If you failed to make the cut-off time, you were eliminated and extracted out of the desert. These deadlines were quite generous and not hard to get inside but were nonetheless a good safety feature to protect people who were really suffering. The long double-marathon stage had a cut-off time of 6pm on the following day, the rest day. This meant that throughout the rest day people trickled in, with the slowest arriving at the camp late in the afternoon (no rest day for them). By the cut-off time they would have been running, walking (or crawling) for a day and night and a second day. There was a pleasant surprise when the race organizers passed the word around the tents that there would be a free can of beer for everyone who gathered at the finish for 6pm to cheer in the final participant. This was a 70-year-old man walking just in front of a 4x4 vehicle with its lights on driving slowly but at a pace to hit the cut-off time. As the vehicle approached out of the darkness, the cans of beer were handed out. The spectacle of all the participants gathered to cheer him over the line is a strong memory and a social media highlight (as the race organization intended). That unexpected can of beer was probably the best beer in the world.

Sadly, that rousing finish was the high point for this last competitor as he was so completely depleted that he failed to complete the next day's stage. I made a special effort to locate him back at the hotel when finally, the race was over. He had been recovering physically in air-conditioned luxury whilst we were still in the desert, but I found that mentally he was so disappointed that he just wanted to go home. Engaging with euphoria of those who had completed the race was not for him. For our part we expressed total admiration that he had completed the longest stage within the cut-off time, falling into the trap of adding 'at his age'. In hindsight, I understand his misgivings. As I approach my eighth decade, I do not want anyone to comment to me that I do very well *for my age*. I do well, or not so well, but age should not be part of the calculus. I don't want plaudits for being an old man who runs ultra races. I am an ultra-runner who happens to be older than most. A fine distinction perhaps, but important. Admiring someone because they are old, makes no sense; admiring someone for completing the longest stage of the MDS does.

The lesson from a week ultra-running in the desert is that you need surprisingly little food to maintain a relatively slow pace. The body switches into fat-burning mode and even the slimmest of runners has ample fat reserves to draw upon. Taking this lesson into my training, I will run for hours with nothing but the water in my CamelBak®. Running in this steady way trains my fat-burning mechanism and means I will not be subject to an energy crash, which usually occurs from eating sugary food, such as energy bars or energy drinks, that raise insulin levels. The sugar is burnt quicker than the insulin dissipates so that, without another shot of sugar, you can come to a juddering stop. Eventually the body purges the insulin and reactivates fat-burning. I find it easier not to go through such highs and lows by not eating. This has another huge benefit. If you complete a long run drinking nothing but water, by the end you are – surprise, surprise – very hungry. Take a shower when you get home and then sit down for a feast of real food. Eating when you are ravenously hungry is an extreme pleasure which many overweight, inactive people never experience. If you do not go through food deprivation, you are missing out. Dieting is not the same. If you restrict food without extreme exercise, it takes a long time before real hunger kicks in. As an ultra-runner, real hunger can be experienced in the time it takes to complete one long run.

It may be that you want to post a good time for a particular ultra race and maximize your performance. In that case, fuelling as you go, taking care to avoid sugar spikes, may make sense. The following method seems to work to allow a relatively faster steady pace (still slow but less slow). Start the race day with a good breakfast at least three hours before the starting gun, of perhaps porridge, scrambled eggs and toast. Then have no more food, just black coffee, until the race starts. During the race, take no food for the first thirty to forty minutes, so that the body's energy furnace is fired up. Then eat a third of a banana. As the energy system is fully operating, this should not produce a blood-sugar spike: instead, it will go into the furnace to be burnt straight away. As the race proceeds, eat a third of a banana or a third of an energy or protein bar every twenty minutes throughout the race. I have found this to be a good nutrition plan to ensure maximum performance, noting that chasing a time is rarely my intention. This provides quite a high level of fuel, so the downside is that you are not very hungry when you finish, blunting the pleasure of post-race feasting.

For the longer ultra races, fuelling up during the race becomes essential. I am not sure if this is physical or psychological; it's probably a bit of both. Asking the body to run for twelve, twenty-four or thirty-six hours with nothing but water is not a good idea. I tend to avoid the pure energy foods and drinks as these empty calories do not contain the nutrition your body craves. I will carry a couple of gels as a pick-me-up in case I end up completely unable to carry on, but they usually remain in my pocket unused. Let your body tell you what it wants. Upon entering an aid station with an array of foods on offer, what does your subconscious crave? Our bodies are very good at self-diagnosing what they need – if we allow them to speak to us. If I had been told this at the start of my foray into ultra-running, I would not have believed it; but I have experienced it and believe it now. At about the halfway point in a 100 mile trail race in hot summer conditions, I entered a checkpoint. I needed to fill my water bottles, of course, but I was oddly attracted to a pack of ready-salted potato crisps. This was strange and surprising because I don't much like potato crisps, particularly when running. They are dry, crunchy and a bother to get out of the packet. I allowed my craving and took a packet. They tasted delicious. The combination of salt, carbohydrate and fat was just perfect. I now try to listen to my body. Other foods that don't normally float my boat, but which I now enjoy when ultra racing, are white bread sandwiches containing cheese, peanut butter or marmite. Offer these to me for afternoon tea and I would politely decline; put them on the table in the latter stages of an ultra race and I will devour them. Again, my physical body is telling me to eat foods with the nutrition it needs.

The psychological benefits of food during a race are harder to pin down, but food, or thoughts of food, can provide a huge boost to mood. On long training runs, I often find myself thinking about what I will eat when I get home, thinking through the options and planning a feast. In races, chunks of dark chocolate give me a lift; I have a supply of these to munch whenever my morale drops. Perhaps the chocolate also provides something my physical body needs, but it is the mood boost that I notice most. One particular incident is lodged in my memory as a positive memory, in dire circumstances when other negatives memories have faded. I was well into a 100 mile race in the early hours of the morning in the mountains and it was raining. The trails had been slippery and there was no avoiding falling over. I arrived at an aid station set up within one large tent. My clothes were sodden and I was muddy and tired. The usual passage through an aid station is to replenish water bottles, grab something to eat and press on. This time, I sat down on a plastic chair feeling totally exhausted. My two water bottles were in pouches at the front of my harness high up on my chest, where I could turn my neck to drink as I ran. I had fallen forward at one point and both drinking nozzles were caked with mud. I would have to clean them before filling them. It all seemed like too much effort. Psychologically, I had just about had it. The race volunteers were marvellous. They took my water bottles, cleaned them and topped them up. They handed me a cup of hot coffee and a slice of cake. One of the volunteers gave me a long explanation of the cake, a local delicacy baked by a lady in the mountain village. Meanwhile I sat there dejected as other runners came and went. I cradled the coffee in my hands and munched the cake with the words about its heritage in my ears. I can appreciate now they were trying to get me to stand up and carry on. I don't remember very much about that night in the mountains now – bad memories tend to get deleted – but I do remember clearly the face of the man explaining how special this slice of cake was and how much good it would do me. The focus on the cake did a wonderful job of distracting my attention away from the pain and discomfort and I was sent on my way back into the rain and the night. My body needed food and the caffeine, but my mind needed the story about the cake and who had baked it.

I keep returning to this idea of eating after training or racing. Instead of forcing down calories in unpleasant forms such as gooey gels or energy drinks, you can let the hunger build to be able to enjoy delicious real food later. The MDS took this to extremes, as it was an entire week of ultra-running over hard terrain on meagre rations. My body had got used to the restricted calories and had operated just fine without noticeably slowing me down. I was slow, of course, but whether I was even slower I couldn't tell. I had, however, developed the hunger of all hungers.

The final stage of the MDS was short; called the 'solidarity stage', it did not count towards your overall time. We already knew at the end of the previous stage that the job was done. We had had one final night in our temporary desert camp, eating our remaining food rations before heading into the open desert for one last time. This stage took us into a particularly beautiful part of the Sahara, full of high, rolling sand dunes. As we made our way through picture-postcard scenes, I spent the whole day in switched-channel mode, simply soaking up the atmosphere and enjoying the desolation, feeling satisfied and accomplished. Approaching the end was quite a surreal experience. We were to catch buses to take us back to Ouarzazate, from a site to which tourists are brought in order to see, and experience, the 'real' Sahara. As we got closer, tourists on dune buggies were driving around and we passed by large well-constructed marquees with huge air-conditioning units attached. I suppose we were just as much tourists as they were, but I felt like the real deal, an explorer coming back out of the desert and back to civilization. Our simple desert camp had been so much more genuine than an air-conditioned marquee. As we boarded the bus, I reflected that I would miss our time in the deep desert. I would also miss the banter within Tent 119, a random mix of people thrown together by chance at the start. Now it was back to normal – and time to satisfy my hunger.

Arriving at the luxury hotel in Ouarzazate, the priority was to reclaim my wheelie bag, which I had not seen since arrival, go to my room and shower. Although I scrubbed myself, the first shower would not be enough. The filth was so deeply engrained that I would not look and feel properly clean until a second, longer, shower later that day. I may also have been guilty of wanting to be quick. An all-you-can-eat buffet was waiting downstairs and hunger was driving my haste. It would be dull to relate the full extent of the hoggery and the number of times I went back for more. One memory has stuck with me. Amongst this debauched feast, one runner stood out. He was loading up from the dessert area, well stocked with a huge variety of cakes and cream and whatever you might desire. There were small plates stacked up beside this area but many of us decided that dinner plates had better capacity. This particular runner had gone a stage further and picked up one of the dessert serving plates with what was left of that pudding, before filling it with pieces of the other options. Having caught my attention, I watched as he walked slowly towards his table, sat down, and proceeded to work his way through this enormous pile of dessert. This would normally be a very rude way to behave, but I could see from how he was walking that his feet must have been completely trashed. When every step is painful, minimizing walking makes sense, even if it is just to the buffet table and back. I could also identify with the degree of hunger he was seeking to satisfy. My multiple visits to the pudding area with my main course plate, first to sample them all, and then going back to load up on those I most liked, was just as greedy but not quite so obvious.

As I think about my fascination with ultra-running and my love of eating, the two go together so well. I cannot help myself from comparing this with another activity which people commonly undertake in retirement – exploring the world by cruise ship. I have not tried one, so do not have direct knowledge, but people report good experiences. They say that the food is great and return home a few kilograms heavier than when they embarked. I can imagine that, with so much good food on offer, I too would tuck in, but cruising is a relatively sedentary activity and it is unlikely that anyone is truly hungry between one meal and the next. I think I would rather spend a week in the desert and then be able to experience the extreme pleasure of eating well whilst truly hungry, and arrive home 3 kg lighter.

CHAPTER 8

WATER IS THE ESSENCE OF LIFE

Water imbalance is crippling,
and dangerous if not corrected.

The risks of dehydration and heat stroke are familiar to most runners. The need to drink sufficiently and often, particularly in hot weather, is standard racing practice. For relatively short running races, such as marathons, the regular water stations provide enough water that you do not need to carry any on your person. For ultra-races, the distance between aid stations can vary between 10 and 20 km, or further. This means it is necessary to carry water in bottles or a backpack bladder to be refilled through the course of the race. Ultra race regulations often require a minimum supply of water to be carried, of between one and two litres, depending on conditions. Most ultra-runners are generally good at following advice to drink as they run to stay hydrated. It is well known that dehydration can be dangerous, and steps are taken to prevent it by both race organizers and runners. What is much less known is that over-hydration is also dangerous, perhaps more so because it is so unexpected.

In my home country of the rain-swept United Kingdom, we tend to take water for granted. This indifference to its importance was nearly my undoing on two occasions when poor decisions caused extreme water imbalance. It is better to learn, understand and implement good water management in advance because to learn by experience, as I did, feels absolutely dreadful.

One place where water is certainly not to be taken for granted is in the Sahara. Without appreciable rainfall, water is available only from underground reservoirs accessed by water well or borehole. The small communities living in the desert are located where there is a reliable water well, and these are few and far between. Running across the desert for a week during the heat of the day with temperatures exceeding 40°C, water was absolutely vital. The MDS race organizers provided water-supply points offering 1.5-litre bottles of water carrying the brand of a local company that was sponsoring the event. Recognizing that electrolyte depletion could be a problem, every participant was provided with salt tablets together with guidance as to how to take them to keep pace with the amount of water drunk. In addition, at the end of each stage, you collected a pack of 1.5-litre bottles to use for drinking, cooking and washing.

This careful rationing of water is in stark contrast with some other multi-day ultra events, such as the Cape Wrath Ultra. This eight-day 400 km race takes place in Scotland over remote and rugged terrain. There was no need to wait for an aid station (which were few and far between) as you could fill your water bottles from the crystal-clear mountain streams along the way. If there was a problem with water, it was overabundance, given persistent rainy weather and waterlogged terrain. In the desert, the situation is reversed, reminding us of the importance of water when you don't have enough of it.

Part of the routine at the end of each stage of the MDS was to wash. You are wearing the same clothes for the whole week. In theory you could pack and carry a change of clothes, but no one would be quite so daft. I had one spare pair of socks, but that was all the additional wardrobe I carried. My routine was to head out into the desert away from the camp with one of my bottles of water and strip off all my clothes. Although there were no places to hide, I put some distance between me and the camp and faced out into the desert to limit what might be on view to just my white behind. I would then wash sparingly with water from a bottle to get rid of the worst of the filth, and particularly the salt from dried sweat. For my clothes, the most critical items were underpants and socks. I would soak these in what was left from the bottle of water and wring them out. Putting back on my shorts and vest, I would stroll back to the camp and hang the wet items of personal clothing on the tent guy ropes to dry. This did not take long in the dry desert air, so the time spent without underwear was short. Feeling a bit fresher, my attention would then turn to eating slowly our meagre rations and drinking more water to refuel and rehydrate.

During the running stages of the MDS, drinking enough water is crucial to avoiding dehydration. This can lead to heat stroke, a potentially dangerous medical condition. This I knew about, and had experienced, years before on a short working trip to the tropics. The schedule was tight and the opportunities to go running were limited. I swapped one lunch for a run, which meant running in the midday sun. This was without any acclimatization; I was not wearing a hat; and did not carry water. Those who are familiar with running in hot conditions will realize how foolish I was. The expression that 'only mad dogs and Englishmen go out in the midday sun' comes to mind. I was not only feeling terrible immediately after the run, but the feeling of being completely pole-axed persisted. When I returned to the UK a few days later, I went to the doctor who diagnosed heat stroke. I was not recovered fully for weeks afterwards. Remembering this incident, the risk of dehydration was uppermost in my mind during the MDS.

General guidance as to how often and how much to drink is of little value, as everyone is different in how much they sweat and how well they acclimatize to hot conditions. One piece of advice I had read in a running magazine was that when you feel thirsty, it is already too late. You therefore need to drink before you feel thirsty. Therein lies a problem. How is it possible to gauge the correct amount to drink to retain a healthy water balance in the body, if you are not relying on your thirst to tell you?

For short running events, there are simple strategies that work. In the military, I served in the jungle of Belize in central America for a six-month tour of duty. Whenever we were in camp, I ran daily at dusk when it was cooler but before it got dark. The circular nine-mile route was a rough stony track with no short-cut options. I adopted an approach to stay hydrated involving drinking a pint of water before setting off. This would slosh around in my stomach for the first few miles. Having sweated profusely during the run, when I returned to camp I would quickly down two pints of water. This somewhat brutal hydration regime worked at the time but I was not tuning into what my body needed. Approaching longer runs with such Neanderthal hydration would have been dangerous.

There is a better way. Before my enforced retirement from racing triathlon due to injury, a top Ironman triathlete shared with me his perspective on the water conundrum. He told me to think of my body as a bucket with a lid fixed on it so you can't see inside. All it has is an overflow hole near the top. During the race, the level of water in the bucket is reducing as you sweat. So, you top it up by drinking, but there is no visible level marker so you don't know how much to drink. The only way to be sure that the bucket remains filled is to drink sufficient to make the bucket overflow. The rule is to drink until you pee; this works well but is inconvenient. In triathlon I discovered an unpleasant truth. The 120 mile bike section of an Ironman race is between five and seven hours depending on your ability. Applying the drink-until-you-pee rule means you will need to urinate. When you are running, you can peel off to the side of road and relieve yourself without losing much time. To stop your bike, get off it, move to side, urinate, get back on the bike and get back up to speed takes an age. Anyone who wants to win a place or set a fast time, doesn't do it. You can risk dehydration by restricting what you drink, or pee in your cycling shorts. The latter is the safer choice. In hot weather when you are drenched with sweat, the spectators do not notice the yellow fluid dribbling over your bike and onto the ground. To the athlete there is some discomfort, but no time lost. To apply this water-balance tactic in ultra-running, you need to keep drinking to ensure that every few hours or so you need to stop for a pee – off to a secluded spot to the side of the route, of course.

On each stage of the race across the Sahara there were regular water resupply stations, where each runner was provided with a 1.5-litre bottle of water. I developed an efficient way to replenish my supplies. I carried 1.5 litres of water in two water bottles, each of 0.75 litres, in pouches high up on the front of my backpack harness. These had plastic pipes coming out of the top to let me drink whilst running. It would look ridiculous to wear such a contraption whilst out running in European climes, but in the desert was a highly practical solution. Pictures of people participating in the MDS almost universally feature such strange water-supply equipment. On the approach to a water resupply point, I would drink whatever was left in these two bottles, so when I was handed my 1.5-litre bottle of water, I could immediately fill my two water bottles. If I remembered, I would also wash down a salt tablet before discarding the big bottle at the supply point. I was already breaking what I now know to be the golden rule of good hydration, which is to drink only what your body needs. I was drinking 1.5 litres of water between each water supply point without listening to my body. We were running through the heat of the day sweating profusely in air so dry that sweat was evaporating almost immediately. This provided very effective cooling but also a high rate of water loss. For the stages that completed in daytime, my water routine seemed to be fine. My behaviour was driven by my concern about the risk of dehydration. I didn't get dehydrated, so my method worked in this regard, but I was still not really tuning into what my body needed.

As mentioned above, the flipside to dehydration is over-hydration. Fortunately, I had read an article on the issue some years before racing across the Sahara. It was about inexperienced joggers running in races in cool European weather and following advice to drink plenty of water. The unusual problem reported was water poisoning. How water could be a poison seemed very odd to me, so I had given the magazine article little attention. Even so, the symptoms of over-hydration had been logged in my long-term memory.

A dangerous situation developed through the longest stage of the Sahara race. I was very slow to realize that I had become over-hydrated, which meant I was very slow to do anything about it. We had begun early in the morning, racing through the heat of the day and into the night. The chances are that, during the heat of the day, my body did indeed need the amount of water I was ingesting. The midday sun had searing intensity, and the air temperature exceeded 40°C. Towards the evening, as the sun was setting, I reached a water supply point offering two big 1.5-litre bottles of water, in anticipation of a longer stretch until the next water supply point. I had already drunk my two personal water bottles on the way into the checkpoint. In hindsight, at this point I would have been fully hydrated, perhaps even on the verge of over-hydrated. I duly used one of the large bottles to replenish my own water bottles. I could see some runners leaving from the checkpoint carrying the additional 1.5-litre water bottle. I didn't want to do that. As we couldn't discard any rubbish in the desert, I would have had to carry it until the next checkpoint, some way off. My not-so-bright idea, after refilling both my personal bottles, was to drink as much of the second 1.5-litre bottle as I could. I probably managed about one litre. My thinking at the time was focussed on the risks of dehydration and, despite a stomach very full of water, I assumed I would sweat it out.

I still hadn't realized there might be a problem. Evening had now fallen, and although the desert is incredibly hot during the day, it is relatively cool at night and can feel quite cold in comparison. I was no longer sweating as we started a long gruelling stretch over soft sand dunes. The water sloshing in my stomach was a nuisance but I thought nothing of it. I then started to feel ill and not just physically tired. My head start to hurt, which developed into an excruciating headache. I also noticed that my hands were swelling up. This was exceedingly unusual and unexpected. I was by then feeling absolutely dreadful. If there had been a way of dropping out at that point, I would have taken it. I was in the desert at night between checkpoints with other runners around, but otherwise feeling very alone. Oddly, I was continuing with the habit which had become engrained from previous days in the desert to take regular sips of water. Finally, the article lodged deep in my memory came back to me, raising the thought that maybe I was over-hydrated. I went over the symptoms of splitting headache and swollen hands, and thought back to the additional litre of water I had forced down late afternoon. I had to laugh quietly to myself. Over-hydration in the desert, what an idiot. This moment of incongruous humour provided a brief respite from my desperation. I still felt so bad that I did not want to carry on (but overcoming such negativity is part of the challenge of ultra-running). I concluded that I must stop drinking. I walked with my head throbbing, unable to entertain the idea of running. I could put up with feeling dreadful because

I knew my body was trying to restore a safe water balance. Each time I stopped to urinate, I regarded that as progress. It took hours before my head started to clear.

It was past midnight before I crossed the finish line of this extra-long stage and crashed out in our team tent. I expected to sleep like a log, especially as the next day was the rest day with no need to get up. But I did not get a solid night's sleep. I was woken many times by the urge to urinate. I couldn't believe it was possible to pass so much fluid. It is only after getting back to the UK that I researched the possible consequences of over-hydration. When the amount of sodium in the blood becomes too diluted, you develop hyponatremia, leading to inflammation. I found information online explaining that, ultimately, the swelling of brain cells will cause your central nervous system to malfunction. Without treatment, you can experience seizures, fall into a coma and, ultimately, die. With this knowledge, I promised myself that in future races I would try to listen to my body and not drink blindly according to some generic advice. You should ingest water according to how much you sweat and, in sustained hot conditions, supplement this with salt tablets. Drinking small amounts regularly, depending how you feel, is the best way forward. If it has been many hours since needing to urinate, you should up the amount you drink until the bucket overflows, as a check that you are fully hydrated.

The year after getting drawn into ultra-running by taking on the MDS, I entered my first mountain ultra. The 100 km race was the second half of the longer full 100 mile (164 km) Ultra Trail du Mont Blanc (see also Chapters 5 and 6), so a taster for what I would attempt some years later. It was a morning start at the Alpine resort of Courmayeur, Italy. The race continued throughout the day and into the night, finishing early the next day in Chamonix, France. It was a brutal event that tested me in so many ways. Part way through, I descended into thinking never, ever again. I came to understand that this was a normal reaction to the most extreme ultra-running events, with such thoughts being erased in the euphoria of finishing. One of the many lessons I took away was the reminder that maintaining a water balance is crucial. I screwed up again; on this occasion it was self-inflicted dehydration.

For this race, in the relatively cool conditions of Europe, I carried two 500 ml water bottles on the front harness of my running backpack (compared with two 750 ml bottles for the Sahara). These were normal water bottles without drinking tubes, so less theatrical. Through the race there were aid stations at regular intervals of between 5 km and 15 km. My habit in the desert had been to drink what was left of the contents of both bottles as I approached a water station. I was wary this time of the risks of over-hydration, having had such a dreadful experience in the Sahara. I was therefore trying to listen to my body, sipping water as required. Over the first half of the race, I found I was emptying on average one bottle between aid stations. This felt like an appropriate balance, even though I had not yet had to stop to urinate. I was too distracted by avoiding over-hydration that I had forgotten the guidance of drink-until-you-pee. In the latter half of the race, in the cool of the night, I was even less motivated to drink water. Up to this point, I had filled the empty bottle at each aid station so I had dropped into the habit of carrying two full bottles but drinking only from one.

At night, tired and hurting, I entered a small aid station to find a long queue to fill water bottles. I wanted to do that and get on before temptation to sit down became too great. The daft notion came into my slightly befuddled mind that I was carrying one bottle too many in any case. I grabbed a piece of chocolate, but did not fill my one empty water bottle, and did not check how far it was until the next aid station. Two mistakes: not filling when the opportunity was available and not checking how far to the next water supply point. One full bottle would be just fine, I wrongly surmised.

I was at the never-ever-again point, at a very low ebb, when I started to feel really bad. I thought back and remembered the water balance mantra, drink-until-you-pee. I quickly downed the last of my water and ran on, feeling no better. I was really struggling and the next aid station refused to arrive. I was slowed to a walk. Although I did not feel the need to urinate, I felt I should, so when I saw that there were no runners close behind, I sat on a rock and tried to relief myself. It wasn't the easiest position from which to urinate, but the little bit of rest for the legs was welcome. Being at night, in the normal run of events, I would have turned off my head torch to preserve my modesty. This time I couldn't be bothered to switch it off. The thought came into my mind of the Monty Python sketch where a member of the King's Court is accused of likening the king to a 'stream of bat's pee'. In response he says, 'What I meant your lord was that you shine out like a shaft of gold whilst all around is dark'. I thought that it might be amusing to leave my head torch on and observe my 'shaft of gold' illuminated by my head torch whilst all around is dark. This slight moment of humour lifted my mood, but only until the flow started. This was not a shaft of gold; it was a very dark colour, so much so that I couldn't tell whether it was red or brown, and more of a dribble than a stream. I was now very worried, as well as utterly exhausted.

The walk to the next aid station seemed to take for ever; breaking into a run was out of the question. I was overtaken by many runners, asking if I was okay. I did not have the shame to ask for a drink, and replied 'yes, I am, just tired'. When, finally, I reached the next aid station, I drank many cups of water and filled both water bottles. I then kept drinking and by the time I reached the next aid station both bottles were empty, and I was not feeling quite so dreadful. I still had not had a pee, so again drank many cups of water as well as filling both water bottles. Finally, the natural urge to pee returned, but with other runners around I stepped off the path, switched off my head torch, and emptied my bladder. I don't know what colour it was, and I didn't much care; I just wanted to survive until the finish. Whatever colour it was, I was not going to let it stop me completing the race. To know might be to worry; better not to know. This is the strange and warped logic that ultra-running instils in you.

How ironic that I managed to suffer over-hydration in the desert and dehydration in the cool of high mountains. It is a fallacy to assume that dehydration is the biggest risk in the heat of the desert, and that over-hydration is a risk only in cooler European climes. The main message is to drink enough, but only enough; in short, to strike a safe balance. This is particularly challenging with ultra-running because so much time is spent running. Whereas in shorter races an imbalance is common and the body can self-stabilize after the finish, in ultra events an imbalance is not so easily cured. Water balance must be managed as you run by being very alert to signs of water stress. An imbalance that is allowed to continue for many hours can be dangerous; remember that too much is as bad as too little. The consequences of getting it wrong will start with unpleasant symptoms, progress to debilitating physical consequences, and can lead to death if not treated quickly enough. Maintaining the correct water balance is vital to safe ultra-running.

CHAPTER 9

DESERT RUNNING

Sandstorms are one of nature's
most spectacular weather events.

There are multiple challenges to ultra-running in the desert, and not just the obvious ones of sun and heat. The conditions can be really uncomfortable, and at times dangerous. The ground underfoot can be tricky, with rocks to trip you up and soft sand to sink into. Sandstorms can roll in with very little warning, completely blocking visibility and making breathing difficult. On the positive side, deserts are some of the most interesting wilderness areas you can ever encounter. The wide-open spaces can be awesome and features such as sand dunes, which appear to go on forever, can be both beautiful and provide exceptionally challenging running. At a glance from afar, the desert seems devoid of life but if you get up close by running through it, and take the time to notice, there are tiny plants eking out an existence. There are also small animals which hide in the heat of the day but scurry around at night.

As I've explained, the ultimate multi-day desert ultra-running event is the legendary Marathon des Sables (MDS). Established in 1986, it has grown from its first line-up of twenty-three madcap runners to over 1,000 today. Its founder, Patrick Bauer, had completed an epic 200 mile walk across the Sahara carrying all he needed to be self-sufficient. He established the race to offer a similar experience to others.

As you've read above, runners must be totally self-sufficient across the 250 km race, with the exception of water, which is provided at regular resupply points. One of the pleasures for me was to be alone in the desert for many hours each day as the initial pack of runners dispersed, each finding their own pace. Where the desert was wide open and flat, you could see the long line of runners stretched out in front and snaking behind, reminding you that this was an adventure shared with others. However, the desert isn't flat, so where the terrain was lumpy and visibility restricted, you could find yourself alone.

At the start of each day, everyone set off together, sent on our way to the sound of the rock anthem 'Highway to Hell' by AC/DC blasted out from speakers fitted to the top of a four-wheel drive vehicle. This was a rousing way to commence each long desert stage. As each day wore on, some runners chose to bunch together for company; I preferred to be by myself. I would speed up or slow down to try to find a space for just me and the desert. I am not anti-social, and enjoyed the company of other runners in the camp at night, but to find solitude in the desert is special. I could imagine it was just me on a solo run across the Sahara. In reality, there was excellent race support with the accompanying safety vehicles kept well away off to the sides to give runners the space to really enjoy the desert experience. The safety helicopter would also swoop by from time to time, another reassuring reminder that it was there if needed.

Desert ultras are to be enjoyed but should not be attempted without careful preparation. Acclimatization is of prime importance to ensure you don't succumb to heat exhaustion. If you do make the effort to acclimatize, you will find that the heat is not such a difficult factor, provided you get your hydration sorted out. This is where I made a big mistake, and I suffered because of it, as Chapter 8 explained. A related and important issue is what to wear for desert running. What might be regarded as 'normal' running clothes, such as tight-fitting Lycra, are not appropriate. There is more on desert clothes below, but first, the pre-race priority for running in the desert is to prepare for the hot conditions.

The body has a slow-acting thermostat that adapts to the prevailing climate. To reset it, the body needs to experience colder or warmer conditions, and this has to be for a period of weeks. You have to force the body to change its biological thermostat settings. I worked in Africa in the 1980s, spending a lot of time in remote places where there was no air-conditioning. My body adapted so well that, after a few months of constant heat, when I found myself in a place where air conditioning *was* available, it was too cold for comfort. Conversely, I remember a member of staff at the British embassy who had been there for years, living in an air-conditioned flat, driving an air-conditioned car and working in an air-conditioned office. She was continually complaining how hot the weather was. She had not asked her body to acclimatize, so her thermostat had stayed on a European setting. There is no short-cut way round this, though: the only way through is to live with the heat and find it uncomfortable until the body's thermostat adjusts to compensate.

In the weeks leading up to the MDS, I wore warm ski underwear, which of course was not necessary in April in the UK, but it helped to trick my body thermostat into recalibrating and being ready for hot conditions. I also set up my exercise bike in a warm space to tell my body to get ready to work and sweat in hot conditions without complaining. These weeks of uncomfortable over-dressing paid off, as I did not at any point suffer from the heat. The desert was extremely hot; I felt hot; I sweated and drank loads, all manageable and safe.

The experience of running in the desert was even tougher than I had expected. Running on sand, as we all know from running along the beach, is hard: sand soaks up energy. Beach running was the only experience I had before arriving in the Sahara.

Aiming to improve my ability to run on sand, I spent time in Cornwall running on the beach and through sand dunes. This was not so much running *on* sand but running *in* sand. It is so much harder to cover distance on soft sand compared with the relatively firm sand down on the shoreline. Without anyone to coach me, or provide tips on technique, I simply bulldozed my way through the dunes, finding it completely knackering. If the whole race was going to be over such soft dunes, I doubted my ability to finish. Fortunately, I found that in the Sahara's dunes are just one of a variety of desert landscapes, ranging from flat gravel plains to rocky mountain ridges.

Once in the desert, I watched how other, more experienced, runners ran, and I tried to emulate them. I picked up useful tactics for running on areas of flat sand and different tips for getting over sand dunes with the least amount of effort. The terrain for which I could not find a good technique were the flat gravel plains, strewn with small rocks. There were so many of these stones that you had to focus hard to land between them. That was generally fine, but you also had to pick your feet up to stay clear of the rocks as your leg swung forward to take the next step. The instinct in long ultra runs is to expend the least effort possible and not to pick your knees up high. Each time I let my guard down and adopted the ultra-running shuffle, I would stub my toe on a rock. The more this happens, the more infuriating it becomes, and the sum of many toe strikes is very sore toes.

On flat sandy stretches, particularly at night, the pack of runners would split off out to both sides. This was unusual, as the standard easy way to run is to follow the path forged by others, letting them lead and navigate. It took a while to work out what was going on. What I discovered is that stable areas of flat sand, unlike the windblown sand which comprises the dunes, have a slight crust on top where the sand has developed a little bit of firmness. The best analogy that comes to mind is running on top of snow where the top has melted a little and refrozen. It does not have the strength to stop your foot falling through, but you get the impression that if you were exceedingly light footed and scampered quickly from one step to the next, you might be able to run over the surface. In the desert the effect is slight, but it did seem to be slighter stronger at night than during the day. This means that it is ever so slightly easier to plant your foot on a patch of sand which has not been trodden on. The landing is marginally firmer too, before your foot sinks beneath the crust into the softer sand beneath. So the reason the field were spreading out was to avoid stepping in the soft sand of other runners' footsteps.

The tip for climbing over sand dunes was completely the opposite. Energy is lost in sinking down into the soft sand. You plant your foot, and before you get the benefit of lifting the body higher, you must expend energy squashing the sand down until it stops moving and gives you purchase. Each step up the face of the dune includes pushing sand down. This is hard work and soul destroying when it goes on for mile after mile. One good solution, I discovered, was to run in the footsteps of another heavier runner. This means placing your foot in the hole in the sand that their foot has just vacated. As you are lighter than the person who made the hole, the bottom of the hole has already been compressed and does not compress further. There is still some give, and it is still hard work, but this is a slightly more efficient way to climb up the dune.

There is no escaping that running in, or on, sand is slow. The positive psychology of such running requires that you forget any preconceived ideas of pace and do not expect rapid progress. Training on my own in Cornwall, I felt extremely slow and dejected. In the Sahara, in the company of other runners, it was reassuring to see that we were all in the same situation. The time it took to complete a 20 km section of sand dunes was more than you would normally expect to run a full marathon. The distance of the longest stage had been a double marathon; in terms of equivalent distance on normal trails, perhaps it was more like a triple marathon.

During the running stages in the desert, drinking the right amount of water to maintain hydration is crucial, recognizing that you will sweat less in the cool of the night. I thought I knew what I had to do – acclimatize in the weeks before, dress appropriately, and remain hydrated. My running clothes were chosen to be cool and minimize exposure to the sun. People who live in the desert show us the best way to stay cool, wearing loose flowing robes that afford complete cover from the sun. I wore loose black shorts allowing air to circulate and long enough to cover my knees. Together with long white socks, my legs were completely screened from the sun. For my torso, I had a very thin top with long sleeves that covered the back of my hands. Under this I wore a lightweight T-shirt as another layer to minimize the risk of sores from my backpack rubbing. My two thin shirts were both white at the beginning but soon became filthy with sweat and blood. It was convenient perhaps that my shorts were black and stayed that colour. My hat was a white peaked cap with material at the back covering ears and neck. Wraparound sunglasses with high UV protection completed the package. The full set of clothes was lightweight, loose for good ventilation, with almost full body cover such that no skin was exposed to direct sunlight. It was not fashionable running gear, just sensible desert clothing. Those wearing tight Lycra and short-sleeved shirts had to be diligent with the sunscreen and had an uncomfortable week.

There is one very special aspect of running in the desert, which is the sandstorm, one of nature's most spectacular weather events. In daytime, they can be seen rolling in from afar, a huge wall of swirling air loaded with sand. At night, the first indication of a sandstorm is the wind picking up (the desert is usually quite still after dark).

If a sandstorm arrives when you are running, you need to hunker down, protect your face and cover your mouth to avoid breathing in sand. Sitting down, curled up with your head in your hands, or lying face down, so I am told, are the best positions to adopt. All you can do is wait for the storm to blow through. When it has departed, any footsteps will have been erased so there will be no tracks left to follow. It is also likely that the marker sticks placed in the sand by the race organizers will have been knocked down or blown away. Fortunately, I didn't need to work out how to ensure I was on the race route in such circumstances. My time on the MDS dodged a day-time sandstorm, but we were hit at night.

Done for the day, we were sitting around chatting under our black hessian shelter. This peaceful scene was interrupted by loud shouting by the locally employed staff, whose job was to move the camp each day to the next location. It was not immediately clear what the problem was. After the initial confusion, word got around that a sandstorm was heading our way. The tent staff seemed to be following a pre-arranged plan. They ran from tent to tent releasing the guy ropes, so that the hessian dropped flat on the ground. We found out later that if they had not done this, whole tents could have been whisked away by the wind. We were encouraged to get under the hessian to find some shelter. This seemed surreal until a short while later the wind picked up to a ferocious strength, with the cutting intensity of a sand-blasting machine. We continued to joke with each other whilst hiding under the hessian. It did not last long. When it was over, we crawled out from under the hessian to find a layer of sand covering the flattened tent. Sand had worked its way into every crevice, even inside our backpacks. One casualty was my sleeping mat, which had been lying loose on the floor of the shelter, but the wind must have prised it away. I searched for it to no avail. It was probably somewhere far away across the other side of the Sahara. The remaining nights were very uncomfortable in my ultra-thin sleeping bag with no ground protection. It hardly mattered, though, as we were so afflicted by tiredness that sleep came easily. If you are an insomniac, try a week in the desert, running long distances on little food; if that doesn't cure you, nothing will.

Whilst running in the desert, one unexpected joy had been sand surfing. A small version of this was going down the face of steep dunes. Normally going down on any terrain involves some effort to control the descent. Going down a dune, you can just let your body go into a sort of freefall, trusting the soft sand to provide sufficient braking. Of course, the fun of this is short-lived because at the bottom you then need to climb up the face of the next dune.

The big version of sand surfing was much more fun, putting a broad smile on my face. It came towards the end of a long rocky mountain ridge with a steep knife-edge hundreds of metres high. The way along the top had been narrow and required close attention to avoid falling down either side. Overtaking was not easy, so it was better just to slot into your place in the line of runners picking their way along the ridge. From this vantage point, if you took a moment to notice, off to the side was a wide, flat sandy plain stretching out into the far distance. This was epic desert scenery. Eventually the race route pulled off the ridge towards the plain below. The way down was very steep and covered by wind-blown sand. It was as if the whole side of the ridge was one gigantic dune face. The runners immediately ahead of me were wading through the knee-deep sand, carefully descending under control. Initially, I followed their cautious example. This changed when I was overtaken by a gung-ho runner going at full pelt, like a skier through powered snow. That looked like great fun. I joined in, leaping down and letting the sand do the work, getting up a great head of speed. I did have a niggling concern about what was under the sand. It was almost certain that jagged rocks lay beneath, given we were descending off a rocky ridge. The uncertainty was the thickness of the sand covering them. I was having too much fun to let that worry spoil the party, though.

My conclusion about desert running is that it can be an unforgettable experience, but should not be taken lightly. The key pre-requisite is to acclimatize, remembering that it takes many weeks to force the body's thermostat to reset. During the event, forget fashionable running gear and wear loose-fitting lightweight clothes that provide full cover from the sun. An essential specialist item is a pair of gaiters to keep sand out of your running shoes.

Prepare well and then enjoy the desert.

CHAPTER 10

MOUNTAIN RUNNING

The 100 mile Ultra Trail du Mont-Blanc (UTMB)
is ultra-running at its most extreme.

Hiking through rugged mountain landscapes is enjoyable. To run through such captivating and awe-inspiring scenery adds an element of danger, which makes it exhilarating. I find being cast adrift from the safety net of civilization, clambering over rocks and running along exposed ridges, to be an uplifting experience. The joy for me is travelling fast and light, traversing challenging terrain and enjoying the raw beauty of the natural world. It makes you feel really alive to be free running in such circumstances, particularly when having to contend with the added uncertainty of unpredictable mountain weather. The pinnacle of mountain running is the UTMB, so tough it almost defies belief. I had not heard of this race before being initiated into ultra-running, but when I became aware of its existence, I needed to know more. The more I discovered, the more I became fascinated by this absolute beast of a race. Finally, my curiosity increased to the point that I considered the possibility of graduating from interested onlooker to active participant. Not sensible, of course, but little about ultra-running is. I was fixated by this race – despite the ostensible ridiculousness of it. I believe that ultra-running in retirement does in general make sense and I recommend it, but I am not sure that the UTMB makes sense for anyone, at any age. This realism comes from the hindsight of actually attempting it. In the years before I took the plunge, I became hooked on the idea and was blinded by the attraction of finishing to such an extent that sense departed me. When eventually I entered, it almost finished me off.

I found that returning to mountain running (I had done some years before) was not straightforward. After being lazy in my middle-age years, I had allowed my strength and resilience to decline to the point where, although hiking was fine, it would not have been safe to rediscover how to leap over rocks and charge down precipitous slopes. This requires your body to take a lot of knocks and survive the odd inevitable tumble. I have continued to hike in the mountains throughout my life, but mountain running is different. Before getting drawn deeply into this special category of ultra-running, I reflected on my brief dabbles in mountain running in the past, when much younger. Two particular mountains are etched in my memory: Mount Kinabalu in Southeast Asia and Mount Cameroon in West Africa. I was not a mountain runner, and had no intention of becoming a mountain runner, but looking back, perhaps these two mountains were my apprenticeship. These distant memories gave me confidence that I could add this special category to my ultra-running retirement portfolio, if I could recover from my slothful middle age, and recapture enough of my strength and resilience.

I first saw the lower slopes of Mount Kinabalu on a bus sight-seeing tour. It was the 1980s and I was indulging in a beach holiday with a friend based at a resort near Kota Kinabalu, capital of Sabah state, Malaysia. The bus trip took in a number of sights, including a stop at the Visitor Centre at the base of Mount Kinabalu, the highest mountain in Borneo at 4,095 m (13,435 ft). Stepping off the bus, you could look up to see the mountain disappear into the clouds. The guide explained that groups of tourists climbed the mountain, staying overnight in a hut beneath the summit to watch the sun rise the following morning. Looking at the spectacular scenery, I wondered if that was the trip we should have booked. It would have been much better than a short walk around the Visitor Centre and photo opportunity before getting back on the bus. My camera had captured the picture, but my mind wanted something more memorable. With idle curiosity, I looked at the noticeboard in the Visitor Centre, where I spotted a cutting from the local newspaper. The headline was about local climbers breaking the record for ascending to the mountain's summit, starting and finishing at the Visitor Centre. The article got me thinking about something much more challenging and memorable than the bus tour.

Back at the hotel, I was getting bored lounging by the pool. I suggested to my companion that we book a two-day mountain climbing trip, but she was not keen. It would have meant swapping a night in our luxury hotel for a night in a basic hut beneath the peak of Mount Kinabalu. To her, that was not an attractive idea. We had seen it, taken the photo and the mountain was ticked off as done. For me, it was unfinished business. My fascination with the mountain grew over the days that followed. I reflected how long it should take to reach the summit and back. I hatched the idea that the record could perhaps be broken. The numbers looked tough, but not impossible. The momentum for the idea was fuelled by my needing a break from the hotel. There is only so much lying on sun loungers and eating buffet meals you can do before you need something a bit more interesting to tackle. The outline idea grew into a plan of action. I worked out the logistics of getting to the visitor centre first thing in the morning and back at the end of the day. I decided that I would head off on my own and give it a go. Impulsive? Yes. Challenging? Yes. Sensible? No. Fun? Absolutely.

Arriving at the Visitor Centre, early in the day, not as a member of a bus tour, I had the full attention of the staff. It was explained to me that I would have to be accompanied by a guide. This was ostensibly for my safety, but no doubt ensured employment for local people. I asked if they had a guide fast enough to go with me for an attempt on the record. I was introduced to a pleasant young man who spoke very little English. He looked fit, and I was assured he was. So, the scene was set for my ad hoc attempt at mountain running. The time on the clock at the visitor centre was recorded by the staff and written in their logbook. I am not sure if I really thought the record was within reach, and I am sure the people in the mountain centre doubted it too. I was not embarrassed to make a fool of myself with people I would never see again. Despite considerable misgivings, it was going to be fun trying and no one need know if I fail. It was more of a one-day adventure to ascend through the clouds to reach the summit, than a genuine record attempt. I was confident of getting to the bottom in time to catch the return bus but there was only a (remote) outside change of my breaking the record.

I set off with a small backpack with water and some snacks, running when I could and hiking fast where it was steepest. The guide–client relationship was reversed with me pushing on and my guide following behind. At one point I took a wrong turn, and he shouted out to summon me back onto the main track. During the ascent, our relationship was strained, as I was pushing the pace and my guide was struggling to keep up, lagging a little way behind. Towards the top we came out of the tree cover and onto a wide expanse of bare rock. It was steep enough in places to require a fixed rope to hold onto. With the summit in sight, my guide sat down on a rock and waved me forward. I ran on alone to the summit, paused briefly, waved back at my guide waiting below so he could be witness that I had indeed reached the summit, and ran back down to where he was sitting on a rock by the path. I noted that we had made good time. We ran down together fast with my guide keeping pace close behind me, as he was better at descending. As we ran down, parties of tourists were hiking up. My guide exchanged excited words in his own language with his fellow guides as we passed. Our relationship changed in that descent. He must have realized that I was not just a tourist with an excessive ego, and that the record may actually be within reach. Arriving back at the Visitor Centre, I was a physical wreck, my legs trashed from descending. It was my guide who was looking relatively fresh, as he explained animatedly to the staff what had happened. The finish time was recorded and compared with the start time. Yes, the record mentioned in the article on the noticeboard had been broken. I asked if some sort of certificate might be possible. One of the park rangers sat at a typewriter and typed out a certificate on headed paper. I handed my guide a good tip and caught transport back to my hotel.

That evening and the next day I was hobbling around, very pleased to use the sun loungers and relax. Subsequently, my record has been substantially reduced as professional mountain runners have attempted it. I was fortunate that it was not yet a record that anyone of true mountain running ability had tackled. I had my short moment of pride, making a rather dull beach holiday something special.

My next ad hoc mountain challenge was a few years later: a race up Mount Cameroon, a dormant volcanic mountain. At the time, I had been working in West Africa and had spotted that there was a race to the top of the mountain, starting and finishing in the town of Buea. It seemed like a suitable challenge, so I had entered, not really knowing what I had let myself in for. The distance was 38 km in two distinct sections: the race from Buea situated at 870 m (2,800 ft) to the top 4,000 m (13,000 ft), and then the race back down to where it started. It was a race of extremes in many ways. At the top, it was cold with patches of snow, whilst tropically hot at the start and finish. The UK fell runner Jack Maitland had been flown out from the UK by the race sponsors, Guinness. He won the race in style, descending as only fell runners can. I was well up the field of runners during the ascent but was much more cautious coming down. I looked at the sharp pumice stone and did not want to take a tumble. I also knew from working in Cameroon there that there were no helicopter rescue services, and limited medical cover. Better to stay safe and not get injured. As with Mount Kinabalu, my legs really suffered as a result of the descent. It would be decades later, when I took up ultra mountain running in retirement, that I finally really learnt how to run downhill.

These incidents of mountain running, as a young man, were individual challenges rather than any pattern of intending to become an expert. The more recent challenge, of racing across the Sahara, was also intended as a one-off adventure to mark my transition into old age. I wasn't to know how this would plant the seeds of a passion for ultra-running. In hindsight, it seems almost inevitable that the allure of extreme running would lead from the desert into the mountains and onto the big daddy of mountain ultra races, the UTMB. The race is 100 miles of steep mountain trails as a single non-stop race. All 100 mile ultra-running races are tough but racing through mountainous terrain makes it exceptionally hard. Like a moth flying towards a burning flame, I was obsessed by the challenge, and it almost killed me.

Long-distance mountain trail running includes the best and worst of times. The routes are physical rollercoasters of steep ascents and challenging descents. The events are also emotional rollercoasters of extreme highs and lows.

The best of mountain running is to feel at one with the spectacular and beautiful landscape. Although when racing, the focus must be on the spot where your foot lands next, there are times when the route is so steep that everyone, except the fastest mountain goats, are forced to hike rather than run. At such times it is safe to lift your gaze up to soak up the environment and marvel at it. Even at night, if the conditions are clear, you can be absorbed by the mountains bathed in moonlight, or gaze down on the lights of small villages below. Part of you is envious, wanting to be inside in the warmth, sitting in a comfortable chair beside the fire and relaxing, but that is for later. The other part of you is relishing the moment, taking in the scenery and enjoying being outside within the landscape, not just observing from afar.

The worst occasions are when the terrain exacts its revenge. The mountains seem to talk to you. How dare you run through here as if it was a race in the park? We, the mountains, demand respect. A mountain route might go from easy running along a track to crossing boulder fields hopping from rock to rock; from safe running sections to exposed segments with steep drops off to the side. The weather might close in, with wind blowing you sideways and rain lashing down, making rocks slippery and the places between into mud. Below the tree line, steep slopes may be criss-crossed by tree roots to trip you up and make a trap for your ankles risking a broken leg as you fall – and fall you do. There is no avoiding taking a tumble; it is how well you land that matters. When the night closes in, so does your mood. Cold, tired and with shaky legs that are struggling to control the descents; this is when the mountains become your enemy. You have to fight hard to continue and get to the next checkpoint. To give up, in some instances would be quite literally to give up on life.

For my sixty-seventh birthday, I treated myself to one of the epic mountain races, the Transvulcania, which circumnavigates the volcanic peaks of La Palma, one of the Canary Islands. The 73 km race starts on the coast at the Fuencaliente lighthouse and climbs to over 2,400 m before descending back to the coast at Tazacorte, with a short final climb to finish in Los Llanos. Although I was hoping for the benign conditions for which the island is renowned, the weather on this occasion was atrocious, with high winds and cold rain. The wind was so severe as participants were following the top of one knife-edge ridge that a runner in front of me took to crawling to be sure of not being blown off. In these exposed sections, I was getting dangerously cold and at risk of hypothermia. Fortunately, parts of the path were more sheltered, allowing me to regain my equilibrium. Out of the 1,000 runners that started, 200 dropped out. Amongst a cohort of experienced mountain runners, this was a huge attrition rate. It was not until late in the race that I descended below the cloud line and felt safe. The mountains did not exact their revenge on *me* that day, but they had me scared.

Once you have shown due respect to the circumstances and battled through, the best of mountain running emerges again. The dawn arrives; perhaps the rain abates; the sun shines through; your mood shifts to positive. Wobbly knees regain their strength. Another section of the rollercoaster of mountain ultra-running has been completed, and you are ready to tackle the next. For the UTMB, it might be to climb yet another mountain pass, having lost count, leading into a second night in the mountains. You must remain in the moment, or the scale of the challenge can become overwhelming. Just another five minutes of running, just another mountain pass, repeated again, and again, and again.

The main difference between mountain running and other ultra runs is altitude. A flat 100 mile road race is hard; a 100 mile off-road trail race is harder; the same distance in the mountains is harder still. Much, much harder. Logistical issues dictate that aid stations are in the valleys, near villages with road access. The race is therefore a series of repeated sequences of climbing into the mountains followed by descent back down, sandwiched between aid stations. In short: ascend, descend, eat, repeat. There is little point in worrying about pace as measured by km per hour; the steep terrain makes such metrics almost meaning-less. The sections that are relatively flat should be enjoyed for the respite they give. More often than not, you are either labouring up a steep incline or charging down a steep descent expending energy to stay upright. Mountain ultra-running has very little easy cruising.

The new challenge I had to master, as I entered the strange world of ultra mountain running, was to work out how to run downhill safely and efficiently. It is amazing to be overtaken by an expert mountain runner, to watch how they hurl them-selves down, letting gravity do the work, and embracing the high speed. Each foot lands ever so briefly as they fly down the slope. I assume that they must take the occasional fall, and when they do it must be colossal. I can observe and understand the theory, but doing it is hard. On benign grass slopes, I try to emulate them, knowing that the consequences of a fall should not be serious. On less forgiving terrain, descending safely and under control takes concentration and physical effort. A set of running poles can be invaluable here.

As noted in an earlier chapter, the use of poles in moun-tain ultra-running is not the same as Nordic walking. This has become a popular activity amongst retired people, to add an ele-ment of upper body exercise to an otherwise gentle stroll. A pole is carried in each hand and planted on the ground in sequence with each step. Many Nordic walkers stroll along the flat with the arms seeming to contribute little to the forward motion. My impression had been that walking poles were an exercise fad which served little real purpose; I was wrong.

As mentioned previously, my introduction to the UTMB was to enter the 100 km CCC (the second half of the UTMB route), commencing in Courmayeur in northern Italy, going via Champex in Switzerland and finishing in Chamonix, France. As

I explained in Chapter 5, Tom Evans, the race winner in 2018 told me that poles were essential when racing in the high mountains. Putting my scepticism aside, I bought a pair and started using them. They still felt to me like an unnecessary appendage that I'd rather not carry, but with Tom's words ringing in my ears, I persevered. It was not until well into the race that I really understood just how useful running poles can be.

On the long steep mountain ascents, the poles allowed me to use my upper body to provide some respite for the legs. As the race progressed, and legs tired, the poles were more and more welcome. I would pack them away for the descents, worried that they would get in the way and trip me up. However, as day turned to night, and I faced yet another steep descent, my legs were giving way. I was having trouble controlling my downward momentum and took several falls. Belatedly, I realized that the poles could be useful after all and took them out. I used them to check my descent and keep control. I hadn't anticipated using them in this way, but they provided welcome stability when descending whilst dog tired.

From someone who had regarded walking/running poles with derision, I am now a convert and would not attempt a mountain ultra without them. My race pair are a fixed length to suit me. I don't like adjustable poles because they can slip and need readjusting, which is an unnecessary distraction. You need to practise using them with different grips for going up and down and different sequences of how you coordinate your movements. I now had the full skill set needed for mountain ultra-running – or so I thought.

Completing the 100 km CCC took over twenty hours, including overnight. I was shattered at the end but through the pain I was also overjoyed to have joined the ultra-mountain running fraternity. The thought took root that maybe I can do this. I now felt ready to contemplate the possibility of doing the full UTMB. The UTMB is not a race you can simply enter as you choose. There are stringent qualifying criteria to demonstrate that you are capable of tackling such an extreme race. As well a medical certificate signed by a doctor, I needed the result of the CCC and another 100 mile race to be allowed the privilege of entering. 'Privilege' is perhaps an odd word to use, but to see my name listed amongst these top athletes did feel special. To even get onto the start line is an achievement. However, that special feeling soon morphed into a worry that this might be beyond what I could manage. Had I got in under false pretences? Would I be found out to be a charlatan?

The UTMB is the ultimate mountain trail running race circumnavigating Mont Blanc, starting and finishing in Chamonix. It is 171 km of mountain trails traversing through Italy, Switzerland and France. Lining up for the start in the late afternoon, there is huge anticipation tinged with trepidation. The centre of Chamonix is packed with runners and their supporters. The race started slowly as the pack of runners wound its way through the narrow streets. Out of town, the road widened, and the pace picked up with runners filling the road. These first kilometres were easy road running, feeling more like the start of a 10 km race as runners jostle for position. The reason became apparent as the race route then turned onto a mountain path heading up into the mountains. This was single file, with few opportunities to overtake. The pace slowed substantially as people settled into their place in the queue. The long, slow line of runners snaked its way up into the mountains with most runners holding the place they had when they turned off the road.

The first 50 km was a punishing baptism into the big race. Late afternoon turned into evening, and evening into night. The field was so large that the mountain paths remained crowded with runners. The terrain was steep, rocky and potentially dangerous if you were to lose your footing. I faced a huge problem.

Ascending the steep paths felt easy at first. On the crowded paths, you just had to keep up with the other competitors. It was so steep that everyone at my place within the middle of the pack was hiking, so picking your way up was hard work but well within my capacity. I kept my place and was happy to be held back a little, as this was going to be a long event taking the best part of two days. A little restraint at this stage would be no bad thing. My head torch was annoying me. It was a simple model, which had been just fine when out running alone at night on the easy trails near home. I found out two things that in hindsight should not have surprised me. First, when the consequences of tripping could be to fall off the side of a mountain, you need crystal-clear vision. My low-power head torch did not provide that. Second, in the company of other runners wearing powerful head torches, I was completely out-torched. It was annoying on the way up to have such a puny head torch compared with everyone else. On the way down, it nearly proved fatal.

The descents were steep, with a variety of terrain including jagged rocks and steep drops. This was as to be expected. The pace was picking up again as runners let gravity push it. I was sandwiched between runners, everyone holding place and maintaining pace. I wrote about this in Chapter 6 in terms of testing my mental resilience but not only was I scared, but I was also in physical danger. The head torches of runners behind me were relatively so much brighter that all I could see immediately to my front was my own shadow. My head torch was drowned out. I took a couple of tumbles from not being able to see where my feet were landing. Again, this is to be expected, but it started to get out of hand. On one steep rocky downhill, we were leaping from rock to rock, focussing on landing each step safely. I fully committed myself to what appeared to be a secure landing place on a prominent rock. The trouble was that being blinded by the brighter lights, I was aiming at a black void, not the black rock I imagined it to be. I didn't just trip or tumble but fell headlong between the rocky outcrops. I landed heavily, knocking the wind out of me. I had no control of how I fell. It was pure luck that my head did not strike a rock. I lay there for a few minutes with a torrent of runners passing by. A number asked if I was okay. I replied that I was fine, and they ran on. I wasn't injured to the extent of needing medical assistance, but I was physically thumped and mentally badly shaken. I thought about how it could have been so much worse. It was only down to sheer luck in terms of the way I had fallen that I was not in need of emergency casualty evacuation.

I carried on, somewhat gingerly, allowing myself to be overtaken. When I was running alone, I was safe and could see well enough but there was always another bright light coming up behind me. As they got closer, their brighter light took away my vision. I seem to be outgunned (or outlighted) by everyone else. No one had a head torch as simple and dim as mine. I had taken perverse pride in not needing a powerful searchlight, but my reluctance to buy a better head torch now seemed exceedingly stupid. Another heavy fall further dented my pride and sapped my confidence. This was frustrating, annoying and dangerous. I had to accept that my night mountain-running preparations had not been good enough.

It was with enormous regret that I withdrew from the race. My mind had been in turmoil. My emotional self was tired and, I admit, scared. My inner pilot was torn between pushing on and the logical analysis that it was too dangerous to do so without a better head torch. I was also thinking forward to the fact that there would be a second night in the mountains when I would be even more tired, reinforcing the logic of my analysis to wrap the race. In hindsight, perhaps I could have gone very slowly until dawn, pausing often to let other runners overtake. I would then have been running in daylight. Perhaps by the second night, the field might have strung out so much that I would have had more space to run without being blinded by the full beam headlights of others. These belated reflections came too late; I had made my decision, and I would have to live with it. I had attempted the UTMB, and it had beaten me.

Back in Chamonix the next day, the race in the mountains continued with the progress of the leading runners broadcast to a big screen in the town square. I felt very low, disappointed and a failure. I couldn't put the letdown behind me. I knew what my wife would say – that she was glad I had got this out of my system and I could now relax into proper retirement. I understand her perspective but that is not my way. My fascination with the UTMB was not out of my system. To stop then would have been to end on a low point; I was not going to accept that. I went around the climbing and running shops in Chamonix investigating head torches and bought the best runner's head torch I could find. It had three brightness settings ranging from normal, through bright, to superbright. The harness fitted securely to my head with the battery mounted at the back making an ergonomic package. I kicked myself for not researching this better and fully understanding the needs of the race. All my night running in preparation had been alone, relying on my military experience of moving silently at night without lights. Although running does need light, I wanted something small and dim so as to retain some night vision. On my own, that was a good choice. In the company of others, it is necessary to have enough light to illuminate the ground in front of you, despite bright lights behind. After the race, reading further about running at night, I found that there was plenty of advice about the need for a bright head torch. I should have sought advice, and accepted it, rather than believe that I knew better.

That time in Chamonix, when I should have been racing in the mountains, was physically relaxing but also a time of mental anguish. To be in and around Chamonix at the time of the UTMB as a spectator would have been interesting but, as a failed race participant, I felt embarrassed and ashamed. Not that anyone was making accusations, except myself. I knew I had failed, and I was determined it would not end here, not like this. Wandering around the UTMB race village, a large area of stalls selling all sorts of high-end running and mountain gear, I reflected. There were now other UTMB events comprising a world series of races using the same format and similar mountainous terrain. Each of these had their own stall with information and leaflets. I was drawn to information about the UTMB Nice to be held in the Maritime Alps. Here I was in Chamonix in the last weekend in August and I could see that the first edition of the UTMB Nice race was just a month away at the end of September. I wondered if it would be possible to get an entry at such late notice. I had just completed 50 km in the mountains, which a month before the race would be perfect preparation for the 100 mile race. Would this be a way to redeem myself, or would I end up as a glutton for punishment with another failure against my name? You will have to wait until the final chapter before I relate how this desperate wish to atone for failure played out.

Both desert running and mountain running are extreme challenges in locations which showcase the best of the natural world. There are times when it is necessary to put your head down and plough on despite the discomfort and pain. It is also a huge waste if you don't lift up your head to notice what is around you and soak up the atmosphere. There is no point in ultra-running if it is regarded as torture; ultra-running in remote locations should be enjoyable. Having tried both in sequence, first the desert and then the mountains, I found the latter more difficult. In particular, you need the ability to race through the night and remain safe. This critically important requirement is where I turn next.

CHAPTER 11

NIGHT RUNNING

It's not only about coping with the dark.

When I held down a full-time job, running had to fit around work. That would often mean training at night, particularly in the winter. Preferring not to run beside roads breathing traffic fumes, one of my favourite runs was along a section of the Thames path. In the summer I would run it regularly, gradually learning every dip and turn, becoming familiar with every trip hazard. So much so, that as the saying goes, I could run it with my eyes closed. At the weekend I could run during the day, but running midweek would be in the evening. As summer turned to autumn, and autumn turned to winter, I would be running in the dark. I would lift my legs a little higher to clear the odd bump which I had not remembered precisely, but I could indeed run the route in all but the darkest of nights.

One hazard to contend with were walkers also on the path at twilight. I learnt to try and make a noise as I approached, or even shout out a greeting. This lesson came from an incident where I came up behind a woman out walking late in the day in winter. I suppose I must have looked like a dark apparition silently arriving out of the darkness. As I passed, she let out a terrible scream of fear. I almost fell over from the shock before we reassured each other that all was well. I still enjoy running alone at night but always advertise my presence as I approach other people from behind so as not to surprise them – or me with their reaction.

I am glad that retirement means I no longer need to run at night. I have the freedom to choose to run car-free routes in daylight throughout the year. However, ultra-runners who want to

compete in the longer races have no choice but to become profi-
cient at running during the night. Entering races that continued
through the night did not initially worry me, as I was already
familiar with running in the dark and felt confident that night
running should hold no surprises. I should not have been so san-
guine. I discovered that there are challenges of nocturnal running in ultra-races that I had not anticipated – and my ignorance
nearly killed me.

Before gaining the freedom that retirement brings, squeezing
in a training run could be hard. On one occasion I was attending
a conference for a few days during the winter. The agenda was
busy, with a short break at the end of the day before gathering
again for dinner. You could lie on your bed; or take a drink in the
bar; or go for a run. Putting on my running shoes, I went out into
a cloudy, moonless night on roads without streetlamps. I could
see just enough to make out the tarmac road. Running down the
white-painted centre line, I could be sure of not tripping over.
Occasionally a car would approach and using the illumination of
its headlights, I could move to the side. There was a path on the
grass kerb which showed up as an indistinct line darker than the
grass verge. As the cars got close, I could jump onto the verge and
keep running. When each car had passed, and it was again pitch
dark, I would return to the security of following the white line
on the flat tarmac in the centre of the road. This was safe enough
as cars could be seen approaching from a long way off. No surprises, or so I thought. I have since discovered that night running
is always capable of delivering surprises, and not always pleasant.
On this occasion, a car approached, and I stayed in the centre
of the road until shortly before it reached me. I was temporarily
blinded by the full beam of its headlights but could just about
make out the black line of the footpath on the verge. Without
breaking stride, I leapt sideways across onto what I assumed

was the footpath. This part of the road layout was different. The black line feature here was a ditch – a deep one. It was also full of brambles. I suspect the car driver didn't even notice me as I launched myself off the tarmac road to what I thought was the safety of the path. It was a surprise as I dropped further than I expected into the ditch, and out of the car driver's line of sight. It took me a few moments to understand my predicament as the car continued on its way. I do not blame the driver because I would have disappeared from view before being caught in the headlights. Pitch dark returned so I had to make my way out of the muddy ditch, extracting myself from brambles, without the benefit of seeing what I was doing. I arrived for dinner late and very much the worse for wear with the embarrassment of fresh scratches on my face, gently weeping blood. When I had the chance to explain, my explanation that I had been out running did not sound convincing. I wondered what the other delegates really thought I had been up to.

My propensity to run in the dark without lights came from my time in the military. Serving in front-line units requires that you be familiar with operating at night without giving away your position. It becomes second nature to move slowly and silently over any type of terrain, not advertising your presence. This became deeply ingrained in my mind as the correct way to travel through remote places. If you were to show a light, you could be seen by the enemy and become a target. If you can move at night without lights, you become the hunter. Even now, when I am hiking at night, I will carry a head torch but avoid switching it on. To me, hiking enveloped in darkness and invisible to others feels safe. Hiking in the dark using a torch feels very exposed. There could be anything, or anyone, out there beyond the pool of light from my torch. My presence is very obvious to anyone who might be lurking, whilst they can choose to remain hidden from me. I find it very odd when people walk through places where there might be dodgy people, shining a torch and feeling more secure because of it. They would probably find it equally odd that I feel safer in total darkness.

Hiking without using a torch also means that you become much more alert to your surroundings. When the sky is clear and there is a full moon, and your eyes have adjusted to the dark, it seems like daylight but without the colours. Getting caught in a bright light, you lose your night vision, extinguishing the night-time ambience of the natural world. For a while you are blind. You then have a choice, to continue by the light of bright artificial light or wait until your night vision returns. An army trick, if you need to use a torch – for example, to consult a map – is to keep one eye closed so you retain night vision in that eye.

Military memories of the night are generally not pleasant, because of the nature of the mission. Beyond the military, being outside at night can be an entirely positive experience, enjoyed best without light pollution. The night in remote places, lit only by natural light of the moon and the stars, is magical. One of my strongest memories of the night time in remote places is from Africa. I was working as a land surveyor in a remote region which, in the wet season, would become a swamp. On this occasion, it was towards the end of the dry season and the surface had been baked hard by the sun to a depth of 20 to 30 cm. It was strong enough to take the weight of my Land Rover, but it was disconcerting when you encountered a weaker spot. The vehicle could break through the crust of hard mud and then bury itself up to the axles. We would have to unload all our survey equipment and spend a lot of time and effort to dig it out and move on to a place with a firmer crust. This would be followed by carrying the equipment back to the vehicle and reloading. There was a slight tension because the rains could come any day, and if they did, we would be completely stranded. We must have been 50 miles from the nearest road or settlement looking out across the dead flat plain, parched dry by the scorching sun. At night, it was pleasantly warm and so dry that it was free of any flying bugs. I was lying on a camp bed wearing only shorts before dropping off to sleep. I gazed up through crystal clear air with absolutely no artificial lights anywhere nearby. The jet-black sky was crammed with stars. I felt like I was on top of the world surfing through the Milky Way. Nights like this, in the middle of nowhere, are special.

I was introduced to running with a head torch through dabbling in night orienteering. This entails running through rough terrain looking for controls. To run in the dark a torch is needed for two purposes: first, to avoid trip hazards as you run; and second, to locate and correctly identify the markers. In orienteering you are not generally following closely behind another runner, and it would be frowned upon if you did. You are required to navigate your own way around the course. I found that a simple low-powered head torch cast a pool of light on the ground in front sufficient to avoid tripping, enough to confirm control identification, and not so bright as to destroy night vision. I felt confident that this was all I needed to ultra-run at night.

To experience night-time ultra-running, I entered a night event. This was the 84 km ultra trail race in Northern Finland that follows the route of the Karhunkierros (or Bear Trail), also mentioned in Chapter 6. The hiking route goes through wonderful examples of Arctic wilderness which can be enjoyed at leisure over a number of days. There are simple huts in which to stay along the way located in delightful locations by lakes or rushing white water rapids. When hiking the Bear Trail alone, you are advised to attach a small bell to your backpack. Bears generally will keep away provided they are not surprised. The small tinkling sound of the bell is enough to warn them of your presence. The incident of surprising a woman out walking, mentioned above, comes to mind. The danger of moving silently is that you might surprise a bear or inadvertently come between a mother bear and her cub. Bears have killed lone runners from time to time, but I was confident that they would keep well away from a whole pack of ultra-runners.

The race start time was 9pm, with the winner finishing early the next day. This was no leisurely tourist hike but something much more ambitious. As this was above the Arctic Circle in late May, the night was short; even at midnight it was not fully dark. Most of the time I did not need to switch on my head torch. There were occasions within the forest, where the ground was criss-crossed with roots, that the head torch was useful but mostly it was unnecessary. This confirmed my view that my simple head torch was all I would need.

The thought that had kept me motivated towards the end was whether I could make it to the finish in time to catch the end of my hotel's breakfast. I know this sounds ridiculous, but reflecting on the dishes offered in a good breakfast buffet was a great distraction from the soreness and tiredness of ultra-running. In the end, hanging around at the finish was the more interesting experience, so I missed breakfast in any case. I crossed the finish line together with a group of much younger runners, having traded places throughout the night. I was delighted that they chose to high-five me as we crossed the finish line. When you are old, and young people treat you as an equal, it feels good.

I took away two lessons from the night on the Bear Trail, both of which proved to be wrong. First, running at night is a breeze. Second, my trusty old orienteering head torch was up to the task. It turned out that the easy conditions of an Arctic summer night were not representative of what I would face in the high mountains at night in bad weather. My existing head torch, which had served me so well when running alone, was no match for the powerful modern head torches now used by most ultra-runners.

In the previous chapter on mountain running, I had to admit to failing at my first attempt at the 100 mile UTMB. I was scuppered by my inability to run safely through the mountains at night. It was now five years on from celebrating my sixtieth birthday in the Sahara, and having reached retirement age, I could have called it a day. No one would have begrudged me that. The problem was that I knew I had failed, and it hurt. When I stop ultra-running, I want it to be on my terms to finish on a high. My ignominious exit from the mountains hung heavy on my conscience and I was determined to bounce back.

After my first attempt at the full format UTMB, I worked hard to correct my night running deficit. I was now the owner of a top-of-the-range running head torch. I wore it out running at night on the trails and through the woods near to where I live. The bright beam felt excessive but if that was what I needed, so be it. I replaced my previous overconfidence with training, solid preparation and good equipment.

I embraced the opportunity to have another go at the biggest challenge in mountain running. The organization that runs the original UTMB race has established a series of mountain races in the same format but different locations. One of these runs the length of the Maritime Alps in France, and through the Mercantour National Park, finishing at Nice on the Mediterranean Coast. For the first edition of this epic race in 2022, entries were encouraged from people with the necessary ultra-running experience. I had the necessary results in long ultra races but one potential problem for me was the requirement for an up-to-date medical certificate. I mentioned

in Chapter 4 how after the MDS, I had been invited to participate in medical research into the heart health of long-distance
athletes. Although I remained symptom-free, the detailed scans
had given the researchers reasons for concern, which they had
communicated to my doctor. When I approached my doctor to
sign the official form certifying that I was medically fit to run
100 miles non-stop through mountainous terrain, he gave me a
long searching look. He asked me why I would want to continue
with extreme ultra-running in these circumstances, *particularly
at my age*. Those words got my back up, but he was right to question whether it was sensible. Of course, entering the full UTMB
is not sensible. I wasn't sure what to reply; I must have replied
something positive about wanting the challenge. Finally, I persuaded my doctor that I would be likely to survive, and he bowed
to my enthusiasm by signing the certificate. I paid the entry fee
and booked the flights and accommodation, all on the cheapest
nonrefundable basis. This was not only to afford it on my pension, but also to remove any possibility of changing my mind. As I
made the arrangements, I didn't think too deeply about what this
would require of me. Once it was all booked and no turning back,
I did pause to reflect, wondering what I had let myself in for.

There are many aspects of this brutal 100 mile mountain race,
lodged in my memory as a series of extreme experiences. There
is nothing to compare with the scale and severity of the UTMB.
In this chapter, I will focus on the particular theme of running
through mountainous terrain at night. To many people, the
whole concept of running in mountains at night is not sensible
or normal. As I write this chapter, I have been reading about the
71-year-old billionaire founder of the high-street fashion chain
Mango, who died whilst out walking in the Montserrat mountain range in Spain. Only a few years older than me, and walking
in good weather in daylight, he had fallen into a 150-metre-deep

ravine. It must have been a sad day for his family, particularly his son who had accompanied him on the hike, but his last memory will be of wonderful scenery enjoyed in good company. This news report makes me reflect on running, at night, in bad weather, and whether that is a good idea or not. The answer, of course, is that it isn't; but nothing about ultra mountain running is sensible. Perhaps that is the point. You do it because it makes you feel alive, really alive, until …

The UTMB Nice race started at midday in the mountain village of Auron, which in the winter is a ski resort. The weather was perfect for running – sunny and pleasantly warm – but perhaps gave a false sense of what might be ahead. The first marathon distance was slow going because of the extreme terrain but it was in daylight, so straightforward hard graft. I avoided thinking forward, knowing that I would need to run three further marathons before the finish. I also knew from the weather forecast that a storm was rolling in, so for the first night of the race there would be atrocious weather to contend with as well as the darkness. I didn't allow such worries to spoil the enjoyment of the mountains at their benign best whilst running in good weather and in daylight. As is typical of mountain weather, the situation did change rapidly from benevolent to malevolent, as the predicted storm arrived with a vengeance. I put on my wet weather gear of hooded jacket and long waterproof trousers. I don't like wearing waterproof trousers, so I had an ultra-light pair which satisfied race scrutineers, although I hadn't expected to ever use them. They were on the mandatory kit list and I had them in my pack but I had never worn them. Again, bad preparation. The weather was so bad I needed them, but they were uncomfortable and annoying in that they didn't want to stay up. I had to regularly hitch them back up. I must have looked more like an old tramp caught in the rain rather than an ultra-runner competing in a race.

Afternoon turned to evening, and evening turned into night, as the storm intensified. Provided I kept moving, I was keeping warm. The going was tough and tiring as I expected, with the wind and rain lashing around me. I had on my excellent head torch which had three brightness settings. The dimmest setting was fine for most of the time, particularly when grinding uphill. This setting also had the longest battery life. The medium setting was good for general running. The brightest setting was for steep downhills in close proximity to other runners, where it is important to see clearly where each foot would land. The bright setting had only a few hours' battery life so had to be used sparingly. Using the full-beam setting, I could see into the shadows cast by other runners' head torches, so I could run with confidence.

The scene was now set for the most dangerous situation I have encountered in ultra-running. First, it was night with poor visibility. Second, the weather was atrocious. Third, the descent was steep with slippery rocks with mud between. Fourth, my confidence had returned. All four factors came together at once and clobbered me hard.

The race route traversed down a steep path. In the dark you could only see the immediate surroundings lit by the runners' head torches. To the right, the ground rose up steeply; to the left it dropped away into black nothingness. The line of the path angled across this precipitous mountainside heading steeply down. I imagined that in daylight, this would be a very exposed path, with beautiful views. This was a path that deserved extreme caution. I had pushed the pace up to this point, knowing that there might be queuing for the narrow mountain paths. I was probably further up the field than my ability deserved and now needed to keep pace with the runners around me. We were all running quickly, letting gravity do its work, focussed on the path ahead. There was little room for error and no additional space to slow and allow other runners to pass. I was in a pack of runners heading down a viciously steep mountain path and the speed was dictated by the pack.

My focus was on the path dead ahead. Realizing the potentially dangerous circumstances, I went over in my mind that if I were to fall, I would have to fall to the right up against the mountain side and not left towards the black void. I had my head torch on the middle setting to conserve battery life and I seemed to be able to see well enough – or so I thought.

The descent settled into a line of runners running at the same pace with everyone keeping their station. I might have slowed down in the wet conditions if I had been alone on the path but that would have held other people back. The consequence of this was that I was running outside my comfort zone. I kept telling myself, if I fall, fall right.

As we descended as a tight group, it became particularly steep and particularly slippery. I thought to turn my head torch to its brightest setting but was so focussed on staying upright that even that small distraction would have been too much. At this steepness, when you slip, you accelerate, and you hope the next step has better grip to bring your speed back under control. If the next step is also slippery, you accelerate even more. This is the situation I found myself in, going too fast, desperately in need of a secure place for the next foot landing. This was all playing out in split-second timing. Fortunately, I could see a black rock, a bit too close to the left edge perhaps, but without another choice it would have to do. I focussed carefully on landing in the middle of the rock hoping it would provide sufficient grip to check the excess speed and regain control. I aimed my foot at the rock, totally committed. This brief moment in time seemed like an eternity. Too late, I realized that it was not a rock. I had been fooled by the shadows. This was in fact a place where the path had fallen away. What I was focussed on was a piece of the black void off to the left. My feet were off the ground, there was no way I could change my trajectory. Too late to steer my fall to the right towards the mountain side. I was falling off the mountain for sure, with nothing I could do about it.

I have reflected many times since this incident that this could have been the end. As I am relating the story, it is not a spoiler to write that it wasn't. If it had been, it would have been premature for sure, but what a way to go!

It all happened so fast, that there was no time to be scared. The fall was arrested almost immediately by a small scrawny tree which was somehow managing to grow against the steep mountainside. My immediate reaction was to grab it and ensure I fell no further. That's when I discovered it was covered in thorns. I had grabbed it so hard that the spikes had pierced my hand. I wasn't going any further down, but neither could I climb back to the path. I was relieved to be alive but also in a state of mild shock and well and truly stuck. A growing group of runners had stopped above me, on the path from which I had fallen. Their head torches shone down on me from what appeared to be the top of a sheer cliff. I kept my attention on them and did not try to look down. In hindsight, I would like to have known what was below but in the shock of the moment I was fixated on not falling further and then finding a way up to safety. Two runners lay down on their fronts and reached down towards me. All I could see was the bright lights of their head torches and two pairs of arms reaching out beyond the pools of light. I lifted myself higher with one or two more barbed handholds to be close enough to reach out and grab one of the hands extended down towards me. It was not so much me grabbing them, but they who grabbed me. Two strong set of arms grasped my hand and hauled me back up to the path. I noted that other runners were holding onto the ankles of my rescuers to prevent them from sliding over the edge. This was a team rescue by the fraternity of ultra-runners. They asked in French whether I was okay. I was conscious, no broken bones and the damage from the thorns not immediately obvious. I replied that I was and thanked them. They were runners; it was a race; they ran on. I still do not know who these good Samaritans were, but I will be forever grateful to them.

I resumed the descent with much more caution. I stopped regularly leaning against the side of the mountain to my right, allowing other runners to pass, keeping well back from the pitch-dark nothingness off to the left. Finally, the exposed descent was over, and I could resume a slow run, trying to recover my composure. It was not until the next aid station that I checked my body for damage. My hands seemed to have leaked copious quantities blood, more than the rain could wash off. A thorn the size of a fat matchstick was lodged in my hand and had to be pulled out, but the otherwise I seemed to be okay.

That incident in the mountains lives with me as an unforgettable moment in time, indelibly etched in my memory as a miraculous escape. I do not know what was beyond that black void. If that stunted tree had not arrested my fall, where would I have landed? There have been accidents in the history of the UTMB family of races where participants have fallen off the mountain and died. How close I was to being added to those statistics I will never know.

The first night in the mountains of the 100 mile UTMB had been spectacular in many ways. It was certainly memorable. The night was capped off with the arrival of dawn. It was uplifting to see the natural light return and the storm abate. I was relieved at having survived and genuinely looking forward to another day navigating through the mountains. The second day was exactly as you would wish in an ultra-running mountain event: abso-lutely knackering. Then, there was the second night …

My ability to recall what happened through the second night in the mountains has been curtailed by blanking out memories best forgotten. My natural tendency to seek peace of mind by compartmentalizing unpleasant experiences has been at work. Perhaps I was so tired that I registered little about what was going on. I do remember hiking up interminable steep paths choked by mud from the previous night's rain. Each step up seemed to come with a further slide backwards, making progress slow and tiring. On the way down, although I was wearing trail-running shoes with extraordinary good grip, the lugs in the sole clogged up and became mud skis. As I approached one control point, the way down was steep with a safety rope provided and race volunteers urging caution. I looked at the trouble runners were having to stay upright, assessed the situation, put my pride aside, and sat on my bottom to slide all the way down the steep slope to the bottom like a kid on a slide. I was already so covered in mud that it made little difference to add some more.

A couple of memories of the second night do stick. The first was my head torch batteries giving out. I found out why the race rules insist you carry two head torches. I fished out my trusty old head torch to see to change the batteries of my powerful main light. To do this I sat down on a rock at the side of the path in an area of forest. The respite was a welcome interlude from the hard slog of moving over extremely difficult terrain. It did not last long; once I had completed the battery change, I was starting to feel cold and needed to get moving. The sec-ond memory I recall is overwhelmingly positive. It was in the early hours beyond midnight sitting down in a tent at an aid station drinking coffee and eating cake. This was not the Ritz in London, Cafe Strindberg in Helsinki, Le Procope in Paris, or any other famous coffee place; it was so much better than any of these.

During this second night, I was tired and sleep-deprived. My inner pilot was resolutely determined not to be beaten, but there was a real danger that my emotional self would let me down. That night I visited the darkest of places literally and metaphorically, the detailed memories of which have been deleted. If that remote aid station with the hot coffee and good cake had an easy shuttle bus off the mountain, my emotional self would have had a fight for supremacy with my inner pilot, with no guarantee which part of my mind would win. Fortunately for my continuation in the race, there was no other option on offer other than to leave the shelter of the aid station and press on.

My views on ultra-running at night are mixed because of the nature of the activity. Night time can be a wonderful experience, but running through the night over rough terrain gives little opportunity to enjoy it. A factor which spoils the potential for enjoyment is light pollution. Within a large pack of runners, the game plays out of the runner with the brightest head torch sees best. You end up running in a sea of bright lights without any possibility of appreciating the subtle natural lighting of the night. I know now that to be safe, you need to play the game and ensure you have plenty of lumens to light the area in front of your feet. I am complicit in causing the light pollution about which I complain. For this reason, I do not find night ultra-running fun. It must be endured so that you can get through to the next day's stage.

To close on a positive note, ultra-running at night can be magical when you are part of a long line of runners, all wearing head torches, extending high up into the mountains ahead, and as a long tail behind, whilst all around is dark. It makes you feel part of a shared adventure. Night running also has the benefit, which applies to all aspects of ultra-running, of looking forward to it ending. What comes next is the dawn, a tremendous positive moment. When the sky starts to turn from pitch black to the slightest hint of grey, you know that the dawn is approaching. It signals the end of a long hard night and the start of a new day. Running through the dawn as it unfolds is ultra-running at its very best. The transition from pitch dark to something less murky makes you look forward to better times ahead. Next, you notice that you can see beyond the range of your head torch, although only in outline and in shades of grey. Your mood lifts as colours return and you no longer need a head torch. Finally, you are caught by the first shaft of sunlight (weather permitting), giving a primeval mental boost as the sun emerges from its hiding place.

CHAPTER 12

BOG PLODDING

Get wet, get filthy, get through to firmer ground.

If you enter off-road races in places where the climate is wet, you will almost certainly have to engage in what I term 'bog plodding'. This is a price you must pay for the pleasure of ultra-running in remote wilderness areas, miles from roads, towns and the trappings of modern life. Accessibility to such spaces includes tracks and paths, which have evolved as people search out the easiest route from one place to another. Such paths tend to follow the line of least effort and take advantage of firm ground. Ultra trail races will incorporate these but also include cross-county sections with no established path. You can therefore encounter a huge variety of terrain, ranging from boulder fields and areas of rough vegetation to rivers and perhaps the most challenging of all, marshland.

The difficulty of some races makes me suspect that race organizers have a sadistic streak which leads them towards deliberate design of the route to be as hard as possible. Perhaps ultra-runners are complicit in wanting to tackle the hardest races, further encouraging the competition for the title of toughest race. High on the list of ways to make a race really tough is to require crossing a river without a bridge or wading through a marsh. Given a free choice of route, most hikers would choose to detour rather do either of those things. Ultra-runners may not have such freedom when there is a prescribed race route to follow, though.

It is to be expected that low ground beside a river may be marshy, but bogs are also to be found high up where the structure of the terrain retains water. Over time, spongy vegetation fills these areas of stagnant water, making a brown soup topped with a layer of moss or grass. To the inexperienced bog plodder, it can be hard to tell where will support you and where it is likely to give way, dropping you into the quagmire. With luck, it might be up to your ankle or knee; if you are unlucky, you could be in up to your waist. The art of bog plodding is to look for a way through, going step by step, reading the terrain. Protruding rocks are always a good safe bet, but these might be few and far between. You can hope also that slightly elevated grassy humps indicate a secure place to plant your foot. If you are following another runner, you can follow their footsteps up to the point where they misjudge and get a soaking, allowing you to switch hastily to a different way through, hoping for a better outcome.

All thoughts of pace, and km per hour, must be abandoned when bog plodding. The smooth, springy stride you might aspire to on firmer terrain is replaced by a squelching sodden struggle to maintain forward progress.

Where an ultra race route follows walking trails and tracks, it can be expected that river crossings will have some sort of bridge. Alternatively, where the route is off-trail, runners will have to choose how to cross water obstacles. This can become an interesting problem to crack. A set of questions may help to solve the dilemma. Are your feet dry, and do you want to keep them dry? If the answer to both questions is yes, you have two options to consider. First, look for a point of constriction where the water is rushing through a narrow gap that can be leapt across, either in one bound or over a few big rocks acting as stepping stones. The second option is to look for a wide place where the water is therefore shallow. It may be possible to run across on rocks that break the surface or are just below the surface, scampering quickly so that, with luck, water doesn't get inside your running shoes. Returning to the original question, are your feet dry? If the answer is no, then simply go for it. Pause only to ensure that you do not get washed away if the river is in flood or a fast-flowing torrent. Some runners have no intention of avoiding a soaking and will deliberately run into the river to wash off mud and to cool down in hot weather.

As I participated in several ultra events in wet terrain, I was slow to learn how to deal with the conditions. I tended to carefully choose my steps making the effort to leap over, go around, or other tactics to keep my feet dry for as long as possible. I know now that this displayed my inexperience. Experienced bog plodders seem to embrace getting wet from the outset. During the Hundred Hills ultramarathon in southern England, recent weather had been wet and turned some sections into mud baths. With difficulty, it was possible to pick your way along the sides keeping out of the mud. This brought you close to other obstacles such as barbed-wire fences and spiky bushes. I persevered with trying to pick my way through, searching out a dry route. This wasted time and only delayed the inevitable soaking. I observed other runners, as they overtook me, going straight through the mud and seeming to relish the experience. The lesson they had taken on board was that there is little point in trying to keep out of the mud. This is a good lesson for a one-day race, where embracing wet feet makes sense, but what if you are competing in a multi-day event? The total impact of soggy footwear for many days in a row could take its toll, leading to escalating foot damage. In the army, soldiers can suffer from trench foot, a condition caused by feet being wet for days at a time. Knowing how damaging this can be, I was keen to keep my feet dry.

I suspect I am not alone in preferring to have dry feet, not just for the reassuring feel of dry socks but so the skin of the feet is not softened by a soaking and therefore more prone to damage and blisters. I have tried several ways to keep my feet dry. One of these was to place plastic bags over my socks before putting on my shoes, but that did not end well, with feet sliding around inside my shoes. Another attempt at a solution was waterproof socks, but they do not let your feet breathe, so your feet get wet anyway from your own sweat. Running shoes claiming to be waterproof is where I turned next. One pair was indeed waterproof but as soon as the water or mud was above the side of the shoe, they filled up. Being totally waterproof, they didn't drain, so I felt as if I was wearing a couple of water-filled buckets on my feet. I should have realized sooner that trying to keep your feet dry is a lost cause.

The issue of wet feet was particularly important leading up to a multi-day challenge in wet and wild Scotland. Entering the Cape Wrath Ultra had been lodged in my mind for some years as a race too far: I feared that the combination of eight days' duration, a distance of 400 km, the mountains and the boggy terrain would beat me. I had signed up to an online newsletter about the race, only to satisfy my curiosity, but in a moment of rash exuberance I clicked through to the entry page and paid the full (substantial) entry fee in one go. I regretted it the next day, but by then I was committed. My search for a dry-feet solution became more urgent.

I located a pair of ankle-high waterproof trail-running shoes and they seemed to work well when tried out on my local riverside routes in wet weather. The combination I decided upon was to wear a pair of thin cotton socks next to my skin, topped by long waterproof socks and finally the ankle-high waterproof shoes. I surmised that it would take some severe conditions to get past this double defence. For the Cape Wrath Ultra, I packed this waterproof trail running sock-shoe combination. Unlike the MDS across the Sahara, for which all you had was what you carried, the Cape Wrath Ultra allowed for a large waterproof kit bag transported by the race organizers. You dropped it off before the start each day and collected it again on arrival in the evening. This meant spare shoes, clean socks and a warm sleeping bag were waiting each evening. I was not sure how my ankle-high waterproof trail shoes would feel through long stages over many days, so I packed the waterproof shoes as my back-up.

I started the race in my well-proven standard racing sock-shoe combination, accepting that it meant spending most of the day with wet feet. The first day was a relatively benign 37 km. Day 2 was a brutal 57 km with a sting in the tail. The final 7 km looked on the map like an easy loch-side run into the finish but was actually a rollercoaster of lumpy hills too small to be portrayed by the contours. This brutal second day meant that I was already drained going into Day 3, and my feet were cut up. One toe had secondary blisters (blisters under blisters) that had burst and were now bleeding. Strapping it up made the pain bearable, but the risk of infection worried me. For Day 3, I took out my waterproof trail-running shoes.

I wore my waterproof shoes and socks for the next two days, taking great care when crossing bogs and rivers not to go in too deep. Water would get into the shoes eventually, but the second defence of long waterproof socks held and I ended the days with dry cotton inner socks. My feet were in relatively good shape, clean and dry.

On the third day of using my dry-feet system, it all went wrong. The route went across another river. Despite searching upstream and downstream, this one did not have a narrow place where you could leap across, nor a wide shallow place to paddle through. There was no alternative to wading into the river. I went for it, as fast as I could, but could feel my double-defences being overcome. I came out the other side with totally wet feet; even worse, water was trapped inside the layers. My system was just as good at keeping the water in as it had been at keeping the water out. The rest of that day was a squelchy, uncomfortable plod. That is the last time I will ever wear waterproof running shoes. It took the experience of the Cape Wrath Ultra to finally expose to me the folly of trying to keep feet dry.

Ultra-running in the wet terrain of the Arctic in the summer is a special case worth recounting. There are extensive areas of tundra swamp punctuated by a few short scrawny trees. The Arctic north of Finland is one such example and the location for the 84 km Ultra through the Oulanka National Park. This follows a hiking trail where wooden walkways have been built to cross the swampiest sections of bog. These are not so much to keep the hikers' feet dry but to protect the ecosystem. Without such protection, hikers would churn up the swamp into a wide path as they tried to find firmer ground. These walkways are just a couple of planks wide and sit on sections of tree trunks sunk into the swamp. They are in effect floating on it. As you run along such walkways, there is a bounce in your step. You need to watch out for slippery or broken planks. If you attempt to overtake another runner, one of you is likely to end up in the swamp, knee- or waist-deep. It is better to hold your position and wait until the route leaves the narrow walkway and climbs onto firmer ground.

This Finnish Ultra race also offered other wet hazards where it followed the path of the fast-flowing Kitka River. The path undulates through the dense forest along the banks of the river, sometimes close by it, in other places climbing up to get around a steep gorge. The scenery is simply spectacular, meaning it is well worth returning on another occasion to hike the Bear Trail at a leisurely pace with the time to really take in the beauty of the Arctic wilderness. Competing in an ultra race, the opportunities to soak up the atmosphere are limited. Along the river valley and gorges, the ground is criss-crossed by tree roots. In wet conditions, the roots are slippery and mud lies inbetween them. Staying upright when hiking is difficult; when running, it is impossible. The key is when you fall, to fall safely. It would be easy to sprain, or even break, an ankle if it is caught between roots when you take a tumble.

Overall bog plodding in the Arctic on established trails is straightforward. The only downside is the need to stay vigilant and focus on where to land each stride. In such interesting terrain, I think it is important to pause and savour the place and circumstances. Losing a little time to look out at the Arctic landscape or crouch down to spot special swamp plants makes such ultras especially satisfying. An example is the distinct shape of the leaves of the cloudberry plant, which requires a very particular location. It grows only in the far north on low hummocks slightly elevated above the swamp. These bright orange cloudberries are a rare delicacy ready to pick in mid-July to mid-September.

Returning to more general bog plodding issues. It has been a long slow learning process to settle on the best method. The general approach to crossing rivers, marshes and muddy stretches is to get in and wallow without wasting mental or physical effort to delay getting soaked. Counterintuitively, the best running shoes for such conditions are not those advertised as waterproof, but quite the opposite. You need running shoes that drain quickly so when running back on firm ground, the action of running squeezes out most of the water as quickly as possible. They also need to fit securely so as not to be lost when lifting your legs from a particularly glutinous bog.

I find bog plodding to be tiring and unpleasant, but a positive spin can be spun by diving straight in. Don't pussyfoot around trying to stay relatively clean and dry; get wet, get filthy, get through to firmer ground.

CHAPTER 13

MULTI-DAY EXPEDITION RACES

An adventure shared with others.

There are a number of multi-day expedition races, including the legendary MDS, which has itself recently spawned other expedition desert races in places diverse as Egypt, Peru and Namibia. In the UK there is the Dragon's Back six-day race down the spine of Wales from Conwy Castle to Cardiff Castle, and the eight-day race through the Scottish Highlands from Fort William in the south to Cape Wrath in the north. Such multi-day ultra-running races are different to non-stop races and require a different approach. Instead of a single brutal challenge, these are extended extreme adventures shared with other runners thrown together for the duration. Join a multi-day expedition ultra race and you will discover a level of tough which makes ultramarathons seem easy.

You can turn up on the morning of a 50 km ultramarathon secure in the knowledge that whatever the race throws at you, whatever happens, later that evening you will be freshly showered and sitting down to eat dinner before sleeping either in the comfort of your own bed (for a local race), or in a hotel or guest house (if the race is further afield). To keep my expenses down for races some way from home, I have taken to sleeping in the car the night before the start. On one occasion I also slept in the car for the night following. This had been a particularly arduous mountain ultramarathon, and rough sleeping after the race had blunted the enjoyment to an extent that I do not want to repeat. After a race I will now always reward my efforts with a good night's sleep in a comfortable bed followed by a huge breakfast. Starting a single-stage 100 mile race is particularly intimidating, knowing that you will be racing through the day and the next night, but the end is still within a timescale that is easy to embrace. The warm shower, hot food and clean bed is delayed, but only by the time it takes to run the distance.

For a multi-stage race, the end of each stage might be welcome for the respite it gives, but it is not the end of the race. Post-stage is all about recovery and getting ready to race the next day. You might dream about a warm shower, hot food and comfortable bed, but such niceties may not come until a week later. The type of shelter provided, and the food available, depend on the race. You remain fully within the confines of the race with no escape to clean sheets and restaurant meals – unless you fail the cut-off time for the stage and are ejected from the race. You are always free to leave of your own accord of course, but it is dangerous to allow such thoughts to gain traction or you might just pull the eject lever in a moment of weakness. You need to be mentally tough over many days to complete the race. The bonus is that finishing the final stage is sweet indeed.

The apparent priority in multi-day racing is to complete each stage in whatever is your best time. The actual priority is to be on top of your personal administration. As an ex-Parachute forces officer, I have been trained to be outside in any conditions, on any terrain, over long periods with only the gear I am carrying. You pack enough, but no more than you need; and you keep it clean, dry (if you can) and in good condition. You learn that poor personal administration can soon descend into chaos. In war, in the heat of battle, you focus on getting the job done and staying alive. However, when the battle is over, the focus needs to shift to being warm, dry and sufficiently fed, ready to fight another day. The same applies to multi-day ultra-running.

The pace you set on any one day relates to keeping enough in the tank for the days yet to come. It is not about posting a good time but about being able to repeat, repeat and repeat again. Backing off on one day, to be sure of being strong enough to survive the next, is part of multi-day racing tactics. In theory, on the final day, you can afford to let it rip, but whether you would be in any fit state to do so, is unlikely.

The end of each day is not when you cross the day's finish line. The stage is over only when you have cleaned up, in whatever way you can. If you are lucky, there might be a river or lake to take a dip to wash off; and the weather dry enough to hang your clothes to dry. If you are unlucky, the weather might be wet and the options to dry out limited. Spending many days in damp clothes is uncomfortable and unpleasant. It may be familiar to soldiers but not welcome when you are meant to be enjoying a multi-day ultra event. In the desert, the situation may be reversed, with water a precious resource to be used carefully. The options are limited to the water you can spare – perhaps a brief rinse for the most personal small items. It is only when you have sorted out your personal circumstances and stabilized your situation at the end of each day, that you can relax. Of course, 'relaxation' in these circumstances is a relative term. Checking carefully your feet and dealing with the inevitable damage is a priority, as is eating to recover and refuel. When, finally, you have sorted out all these issues, you can wind down and reflect on how the day has panned out.

Injury in multi-day ultra-running events is a major risk. Soldiering on through minor injury in a single-stage race is normal. For multi-day racing, every injury, no matter how small, must be dealt with early to ensure it does not escalate into something more serious. Any broken skin, such as burst blisters, must be kept clean to avoid infection.

Feeding regimes in organized multi-day ultra-races vary between two extremes. For the week-long MDS race across the

Sahara, the only food available was what you carried. Post-stage feeding was therefore according to a carefully planned menu with exactly what your body needed, but no more. The race regulations stipulated a minimum number of calories; for many of us this became the target to keep our backpacks as light as possible. To fully satisfy the hunger induced by running a series of ultramarathons would mean travelling through the day weighed down like a pack mule. Better to keep it frugal and simple and look forward to satisfying a ravenous hunger when the entire race is over.

At the other end of the feeding spectrum was the Cape Wrath eight-day ultra through the Scottish Highlands, where food was provided by the organizers. Like the MDS, the race provided a tented camp that relocated to a new location each night. A highly efficient race organization would take the tents down, transport them to the next site and then put them up again, ready to receive the runners at the end of the day's stage. The large team of staff doing this work were led by a few employed professionals but were predominantly volunteers. Their enthusiasm shone out, and I wondered what motivated them. Through discussion, I found out what was going on. The business model employed was that by giving up eight days of their time to join the race organization team, they could earn a substantial discount on the fee to enter future races. This meant they were not just workers but fellow ultra-runners who shared the passion for the sport and understood what each of us was going through. The team spirit of the support staff was so strong that I found that some of the volunteers were there simply to enjoy volunteering, with perhaps a partner who was there to earn a race entry discount. People like me, who were receiving the enjoyment of competing without having contributed time or effort to the organization, paid a substantial entry fee, but other runners who had grafted in previous editions paid much less. This worked for everyone and made for a wonderful communal atmosphere.

A member of the Cape Wrath Ultra race team who particularly impressed was the race doctor, also a volunteer, who was spending valuable holiday time to do a difficult and sometimes stressful job. She was herself an ultra-runner so had deep understanding to match her medical expertise. My edition of the Cape Wrath Ultra race was hit by a contagious vomiting bug, which in the close confines of the camp and shared facilities could have caused havoc. The race doctor insisted on strictly enforced hygiene controls. As soon as symptoms became apparent, the person would be put into quarantine for forty-eight hours. They were evicted from the eight-person shared tents and put into a segregated compound of small single-person tents with a couple of dedicated portable toilets. This reallocation could take place even in the middle of the night. It is to the credit of the race crew that only about 10 per cent of runners were afflicted with the highly infectious bug. I was also impressed that many of these runners continued the race whilst in quarantine and suffering diarrhoea and vomiting. Ultra-running is hard enough without adding such an extra burden.

For the Cape Wrath Ultra, unlike the MDS, there was a kitchen tent and a dining marquee. In cold, and often wet Scotland, this was very welcome. At the end of the stage, the kitchen was serving hot soup and unlimited quantities of chips fresh from the deep-fat fryer. I watched some runners munch their way through double helpings of these, covered in tomato ketchup, mayonnaise or chilli sauce; or a combination of all three. At the end of the first day, I joined in, but a stomach full of chips is not actually what my body wanted. For the other days I stuck to soup and waited to fill up at dinner, which was a simple vegetarian meal, again in unlimited quantities. Having eaten well, I would crawl into my sleeping bag for a long, deep slumber, despite the hard ground and shared tent arrangements.

Back home in my comfortable bed, I am a light sleeper. Outside in the relatively rough conditions of an ultra-running camp, I tend to sleep much better. It may be that being outdoors is the reason. I went back to the location of my 84 km single-stage ultra race along the Bear Trail in Northern Finland with my daughter, hiking it over a relatively leisurely 3 days. This time I could marvel at the surroundings and share the experience with her. We were eating simply and sleeping on the hard boards of the open-plan trail huts. On arrival at the trail end in Ruka, we both noticed the contrast between the beautiful natural wilderness we had experienced along the trail and the ski resort in the summer without snow cover. Whereas in the winter it may look like a winter wonderland, in the summer it looked somewhat shabby and the ski lifts resembled scars on the natural landscape.

We had been looking forward to ending our spartan hike with a night in Ruka, amongst the après-ski bars, restaurants and hotels. The hotel was indeed luxurious, but in the apparent comfort of the hotel, we both found it hard to sleep. Somehow the austere conditions on the trail were conducive to sleeping well. Perhaps it was the fresh air, nature noises or the soothing sound of rushing water, as many huts were close by a stream. Such experiences are a reminder that the coddled world of modern living may not be what our minds really need to be relaxed and content.

An inescapable aspect of multi-day ultra-running is the comradeship. Whether you like it or not, whether you are a social animal or not, you are stuck in a bubble with the other runners. When I run, I prefer to enjoy the sounds of nature and imagine I might be alone in the wilderness. If a group of runners are chatting as they go, which at ultra-running pace for those in the middle of the pack is possible, I tend to either speed up or slow down to put some distance between me and them. In the camp, it is different. I enjoy meeting other people and the mutual support of sharing the same trials and tribulations to get through from one day to the next. I have very happy memories of Tent 119 on the MDS and the fun we had keeping ourselves entertained, without the intrusion of television or social media. If you don't enjoy close social engagement with people that you have not met before, do not enter a multi-day ultra-event.

Once you start a multi-day ultra race, there is no escape from the race 'bubble'. I discovered that although this is usually the case, this is not necessarily always so. During one evening of the Cape Wrath Ultra one of my tent buddies was nowhere to be seen until late. He explained the next morning that he had been exploring and found a pub a short hike away which served good beer and bacon butties. I berated him for not reporting back to his tent mates, but as we were too remote for mobile phone reception, he had a decent excuse. If I had looked more carefully at the map, I too could have spotted the remote isolated public house. The race organizers were not going to tell us and risk the pub being swamped by 100 malodorous ultra-runners.

Multi-day ultra-running is a very special challenge but it's not for everyone. You need to be resilient and able to cope with the long distance, terrain and prevailing weather, as well as enjoy being part of an adventure shared with others. If you can handle all this, you will have a huge amount of fun and log some of your very best ultra-running memories.

CHAPTER 14

LIMIT TRAINING

It's not about racing.

How to train for ultra-running depends on you as an individual, your aspirations, your circumstances, and what you find acceptable and enjoyable. Adopting someone else's training plan, no matter how well designed, is unlikely to work. General training principles are offered here, geared to the older retired person. They can be summarized as limiting training to that which is sensible and not onerous. The specifics are up to you.

When you retire, there are life changes that influence how you train, starting with acceptance that your body has aged such that strength and resilience cannot be taken for granted. This inescapable truth sets the context for considering what training is appropriate. Whilst age constrains what you are capable of, you have the freedom to set objectives that are right for you. Released from the expectations of work and raising a family, you have the opportunity to train whenever you want, for as short or as long as you want.

Racing may have been an objective of your younger self but as you get more mature, that must change or you will suffer. I observe people who continue to race into old age, and they seem to run themselves into the ground. The frustration of getting slower has fuelled them to push even harder. The target becomes to be competitive in the next age-group category, to win the over-50, over-55, over-60, over-65, over-70, and onward to oblivion. In my view, this is self-defeating. As you get older, you need to stop focussing on racing for racing's sake and concentrate instead on enjoying the health benefits of continuing to run. It is not about beating yourself up because your split times are slower; it should be about accepting that your split times will of course be slower, and it doesn't matter.

As I started ultra-running, I was guilty of getting sucked into the racing trap. As I've mentioned, my first big event was the MDS in the year of my sixtieth birthday. The first day eased us into the event with a relatively easy single-marathon distance. Considering the harsh conditions, I ran what I considered to be a decent time. Although my intention was not to race, driven by habit I looked up my position at the end of the first day. My time would have put me well placed in the over-60 category, but my name was not there. I enquired at race control, and they said that my birth date did not fit the over-60 category definition. As I had turned sixty some weeks before, this made no sense to me, but I had to accept that rules are rules. The next day was an ultramarathon, and I enjoyed a day of running without pressure, focussed on enjoying the occasion and savouring the experience of the desert. I had to admit to myself that this was a much more appropriate mindset. Ironically, my situation had been reviewed during that second day such that the results *did* then have me in the over-60 category, but by then I was some way off contention. It is probably healthy that my race was over almost before it had begun. I could enjoy participating without feeling that I needed to race. That is the single most important aspect of ultra-running in retirement; it is not about racing. My personal objectives of ultra-running are to push back against the ageing process and enjoy the feeling of remaining active. Using your body feels good, with a wonderful bonus that eating is much more pleasurable when you really need the calories.

There are some common running training guidelines that are worth adhering to. One of these is not to increase your running mileage by more than 10 per cent per week. Another is the need to stretch and warm up before you run. Apart from these, there is a huge variety of possible training schemes. The discussion in this chapter is about what I have found works for me, without getting sucked into an intense and prescriptive training regime. I want to be healthy, have fun and compete, in that order of priority.

Training for health is based on the principle of 'use it or lose it'. Our bodies are dynamic living systems that respond to what we ask of them. If we remain active, putting our body under physical stress, it responds by staying strong. If we sit and do very little, for days, weeks, months or, in some cases, years, the body weakens. This applies to everyone at any age but is acute as you get older when the ageing process will accelerate the decline.

One example that reinforces the use-it-or-lose-it perspective is the case of astronauts. These are fit, healthy, relatively young people in the prime of life. When they are weightless in orbit for week or months, though, they get weaker. One of the body's many mechanisms is that bone cells respond to stress by getting stronger. The amazing engineering perfection of our bones to be robust and strong exactly where that strength is needed is the result not of engineering design, but rather because of the simple mechanism of cellular response to physical stress. Where the stress is greatest, the bones are strongest. Without the regular physical stress of weight-bearing activity, the fit young astronauts' skeletons lose bone mass and strength. Back on earth, they need to ease back into activity to avoid injury and recover their physical health. The muscular and cardiovascular systems have similar responsive mechanisms.

As your body clock ticks past sixty, caution is needed. Overdoing the training or launching into training from a complete standstill risks injury. Damage could arise from the simple act of going for a run out of the blue. As outlined in an earlier chapter, if this happens and is interpreted as needing to avoid running, you'll actually be doing the opposite of protecting your-self, hastening the physical decline. I so often hear people my age say that they no longer run because their joints can't take it. Accepting that there is a level of decline from which it is hard to recover, the general advice is use it or lose it. If you have already lost it, recovery may be difficult. Yet there is still hope. One way back is to purchase highly cushioned running shoes to reduce the severity of the impact of running. Another is to try running in a swimming pool. If this becomes a permanent alternative to running outside, it will have limited value. If this is part of a transition to getting back into running on land, however, it can be a safe and effective method. This is exactly what happens to expensive racehorses that get injured; they are put to run in equine swimming pools to hasten recovery with low-impact exercise.

Running in later years is about staying strong, active, happy and healthy. The idea, if you buy into it, is to be healthy and active for as long as possible, accepting that the day will come when the lights go out. Running does include the risk that it could cause your demise. That risk goes up with age and with the severity of the races you attempt. Blasting out your best time for a 10 km race does indeed put your body under considerable stress. I have decided that such relatively short races are no longer appropriate for me. I have the mental discipline to push my body hard, but I no longer do so, because I fear that I could blow a fuse. I am much happier to run slow and steady. Ultra-running is hard only because of the duration and cumulative stress of many hours. Each kilometre of an ultramarathon is a breeze and I cannot envisage that this level of physical exertion could be the cause of finishing me off. Ultra-running, I believe, can reduce the period of old ill health. Instead of struggling with chair lifts, Zimmer frames and mobility scooters for years, or even decades, you can stay active until your last breath.

Whether you should follow the guidance offered here is up to you. All I can do is to share some thoughts for you to consider. You may not want to race; you may not want to run ultra-marathons; do only what suits you. I ask just that you reflect on what I have to say, feeling free to accept, reject or amend. What works for you depends on you; this is the fundamental principle of training in retirement.

Let us begin with an important core component of training: rest. It is when you're resting between training sessions that the body repairs and strengthens. Whatever else you do, do not neglect the need to rest. To ensure this, it is good sense to dedicate one day each week to *not* running. If you have an injury of some sort, even a minor niggle, extend this to three days' rest. Don't get frustrated by the lack of training; simply enjoy the break. You should stay mobile – perhaps go swimming – but enforce the no-run rule to give your body the chance to repair. This should apply to runners of all ages but is particularly important for us oldies who take a bit longer to recover than younger athletes.

If an injury does not fix itself within three days, you should probably seek medical advice. A busy doctor may ask why you want to continue running at your age. It is a question I have been asked and it annoys me. It is true that the NHS is under enormous strain dealing with old people who are ill. One perspective is resources should be focussed on ill old people, not healthy old people. To echo my thoughts in Chapter 4, such a system is not a healthcare system, rather an illness-management system. A true healthcare system would focus on keeping old people healthy. Instead of being clogged up with old people suffering long-term chronic illness brought on by sustained inactivity, imagine a system in which the end-of-life window of ill health is short, or non-existent. Running can keep us healthy until the day we drop. Medical advice directed towards keeping elderly people active should be regarded as a good investment of doctors' time. The medical professionals of most use to runners are physiotherapists. Their expertise lies in activating the body's self-repair mechanisms to rehabilitate people after injury. Instead of popping pills, they design exercises to get the body to repair itself. When I have been injured, physiotherapists have recommended exercises that I have collected and which have become part of my regular daily routine. It is a shame that it was only through injury that I learnt about them. Medical experts are great but remember that the primary healthcare professional is yourself, in the sense if your taking responsibility for your own health, in so far as you are able.

Having emphasized the importance of rest in any training programme, you can have too much of a good thing. If all you do is to rest, you'll soon become weak and unfit. The only time when sustained rest makes sense is the week before a race. The pre-race week should include general activity like stretching and short easy runs, as well as swimming perhaps. This is simply keeping the body ticking over and ensuring complete recovery from training in the weeks before.

Between periods of rest, you need to train, of course. I will outline below some thoughts on running training, both slow and fast, and consider the importance of time in the gym.

The essence of ultra-running is to run slowly for a long time over long distances. It therefore makes sense for a large proportion of your training to be running slowly for a long time. These training runs should be as long as you find enjoyable. Scenic routes can help to make a long run a pleasant experience. Some people like to listen to music, although I don't. I enjoy being outside soaking up the sounds of nature and remaining alert to my surroundings.

My long training runs are three to five hours in duration. More than five hours gets uncomfortable, so I save that experience for racing. By racing, I mean in the relative terms, as I don't now race in the sense of pushing my body hard. For me, 'racing' means holding a comfortable pace without slacking off. If you can hold such a moderate pace for many hours, it can translate into a good position in the middle of the pack of ultra-runners. It will not get you up with the frontrunners, but it is enough to put you in contention against other oldies and the possibility of an age-group prize.

What to eat on a long training run depends on where I am within a training cycle. If I am training for a particular event where I intend to post a decent time, then I will nibble on a banana or protein bar as I run. Eating on the go allows my comfortable pace to be a little faster. It is worth noting that I always avoid the junk calories of energy drinks or gels with little nutritional value. If I don't have a race on the immediate horizon, then I drink just water. This ensures that my fat burning metabolism is fired up and has the added benefit building up an appetite which needs sating with good food when the run is over.

Speed training should not be ignored. If all you do is to run slowly, then all you'll ever be able to do is run slowly. Even for ultra-running, interval training improves resilience and flexibility. Hill intervals are good for improving climbing strength, while flat intervals improve your running motion. I do these at the top end of my comfortable running pace, enforced through setting a maximum pulse rate. This limit has come down over the years but note that general guidance on maximum pulse rate related to age is of little relevance. You should work out what numbers correspond to you. One way to work out your maximum pulse rate is by running as hard as you can, holding the pace over an extended period, and measuring your pulse rate. Such tests are for younger people. You wouldn't drive a classic car with your foot to the floor to find out its top speed for fear of blowing up the engine. The same caution should be applied to older human bodies. Explore the pulse rate that matches a comfortable fast running pace, assessed through how you feel. This pulse rate should then be used as an upper limit not to be exceeded. This prevents the excitement of a race, or over-exuberance in training, from taking you outside your safe cardiovascular envelope.

When I was young, my mind was weaker than my body. I could push as hard as the pain I could trick my mind into tolerating, knowing that my body would be fine. In old age, this has reversed; my mind is stronger than my body. I have the experience to be able to push myself through all sorts of levels of pain, overriding how my body feels to such an extent that I believe I could rupture something. I may be wrong, but I do not intend to find out.

Strength training is essential to remain free of injury, even though ultra-running is a slow aerobic activity for which strength is not an obvious requirement. Certainly, a bulked-up muscular body would slow you down, but being strong is needed to cope with the unexpected. Running on smooth, flat tarmac in daylight is straightforward and should not hold any surprises. Running over rough terrain, especially going fast downhill, and perhaps at night, might mean a surprise at every step. Trips and awkward landings are standard, and dealing with them requires core strength so that you can brace yourself against heavy asymmetric loads. I found this out first-hand during training for my first big ultra race across the Sahara. I tripped and pulled a muscle, luckily not badly, but I was concerned that it might bring a premature halt to my big adventure. It was then that I developed a set of exercises to improve my core strength. I would do the set every morning. It became a habit that I follow without thinking. It was hard at the start but years later is now easy, and as automatic as getting out of bed. I feel so much stronger now than

I did in middle age, a period of my life when I had allowed my strength to wane. I figure that if I can do the exercise set today, I can do it tomorrow, next week, next month, next year, next decade, for as long as I live. There should be no reason, apart from major illness, why I cannot repeat from one day to the next. I hope that if I make it into extreme old age, I will still be doing the exact same set of exercises I have been doing for nearly a decade already. The exercise set was designed for a 60-year-old; if I can still handle it aged eighty and beyond, that would be just great.

In addition to sets of formal exercises, regular exercise – such as climbing stairs – can be incorporated into normal home life whenever the opportunity arises. Such low-level exercise is good but not sufficient. You also need to spend time in the gym. The ageing process tends to weaken our bodies. Without mitigating action, as people get older, they will find it harder to run, then hard to walk, and finally succumb to getting around on a mobility scooter. Far too many older people accept this decline as inevitable and even plan for it by fitting a stair-lift ready for when they are unable to climb the stairs. This defeatist attitude is not for me. The alternative is to halt the decline by maintaining regular activity that includes heavy weight training. This builds strength, hopefully at a similar rate to weakening from ageing, allowing you to maintain physical capabilities well into old age. Whether you run ultramarathons or not, all old people should develop a gym habit. Ultra-runners need to retain strength to be able to take the punishment of rough terrain without injury. If you are new to the gym, start easy. There is no point going there only to get injured from trying to do too much too soon; the whole aim of gym work is injury prevention.

Finally, as an ex-triathlete, I keep swimming as part of my training. This low-impact exercise is particularly useful when your legs need a rest. In line with my altered retirement psychology, I do not look at the wall clock to see what splits I am swimming. These are so far adrift from my triathlon days that it would be depressing. Deliberating not looking, and not knowing, is a conscious decision that I don't care. I swim a moderate distance relatively slowly and feel better for it. It is now a very chill (in all senses) activity. Indoor pool swimming is fine, but the real fun comes with outdoor or wild water swimming. I regularly spend time in a small cottage by Lake Saimaa in Finland. When there, I will swim each morning no matter the weather or the time of year. In the winter it requires some pre-work to cut a hole in the ice, but I continue to swim. Perhaps my terminology is wrong; in the winter it is a dip in the ice-hole rather than a real swim. It's still an exhilarating experience that sets you up for the day. Even when the ice has melted in the spring, the water remains cold except for a brief period in the height of summer when the long sunny days raise the lake water to a comfortable temperature. The open-water combination of exercise and cold gives the system quite a jolt. It has been described to me as the body registering a 'near-death experience' by flooding your body with endorphins. It makes you feel great. There is a risk, of course, in the years ahead that if I suffer a heart attack, this might just be the trigger. I therefore swim close to the shore so it would be relatively easy to fish me out. People ask if this is a risk I should be taking. I think it is. Feeling just great until your final day is how life should be lived.

CHAPTER 15

ULTRA-RUNNING AS RELAXATION

Relax and enjoy is the way to race in retirement.

Relaxation and ultra-running may seem like odd bedfellows, but on closer examination they complement each other rather well. Relaxing can improve the way you run; and the activity of ultra-running can help you to relax. There is a grand synergy to be exploited.

It goes without saying that you want to relax in your retirement. Running in order to relax might not be every pensioner's choice, especially over long distances. The key to understanding how this combination works is the distinction between physical and mental relaxation. It may not be evident that ultra-running can be physically relaxing; it's easier to appreciate that it can offer incredibly good mental relaxation. Letting your mind roam free on a long run outside amongst the sights, sounds, and smells of the natural world, is just about the best mental escape yet devised. If you are wound up, tense or worried, then the more obviously relaxing activity of sitting around doing nothing can achieve the opposite. The inactivity allows your worries to fester and can lead to a feeling of hopelessness. Standing up, putting on your running shoes and getting out the door are the positive moves you need to break out of mental stupor. When your conscious effort is focussed on where your next stride will land running over rough terrain, the mental release can be pure joy.

Can racing be relaxing? The obvious answer is no. If I think back to my triathlon racing days, relaxation was not part of the package. In the first few hundred metres, you would swim hard to get amongst a pack of the better swimmers. There would then be a fight to keep your place drafting close behind other swimmers. There could be short periods of the swim segment when the level of effort could be less when slotted in behind a swimmer of similar ability. Keeping so close that your hands were almost touching their ankles, you could be sucked along in their wake. There would be little advantage to be gained by overtaking. It only takes a few races to realise that it makes little sense to move aside and forego the tow, only to be swimming alongside at the same pace. So, you accept your place and cruise, enjoying the brief respite. It may last only until you spot the opportunity of a better swimmer, or line of faster swimmers, overtaking. You then need to rejoin the maelstrom of the race, swimming hard to catch a better ride behind the faster swimmer. The bike stage was even more intense, pushing to keep the average speed high. My riding position on my racing bike was highly aerodynamic but also uncomfortable. This was the price of that little bit of extra pace. On the run, it was all about how hard you could push, how close to the red zone you could hold it without blowing up. Such racing was exciting, not to mention hugely satisfying if you did well, but relaxing it was not.

Ultra-races can, and in my opinion should, be relaxing. I observe the runners who win ultra-races, admire their commitment and drive, but that is not for me. Such full-on racing is not compatible with retirement. Even if you still hanker to race, if you focus on racing in an ultra-run, you are likely to end up losing. If you try to be a hare and dash off from the start, after a few hours you will suffer and probably end up walking. Embrace the fact that you are a tortoise and just keep going. In ultra-races, tortoises can win. The attrition rate on the long races can be high. The person in your age group up ahead may be a hare who later drops out, or you might find that you can slowly overtake towards the end whilst they are so pooped that they have resorted to walking. If you aspire to win one of the older age categories, just getting to the finish might be enough. Relax and enjoy is the way to race in retirement, even if you aspire to do well against others your age.

The mental attitude to take you through an ultra-run is to relax and let the time flow by. Another twenty minutes, another hour, slowly picking off landmarks along the route. Don't be a slave to split times and pace. In the race across the Sahara, although other runners had their hands on their watches at the start of each day to activate the stopwatch function, I did not. My simple watch told me only the time of day, giving me a general idea of how far through the stage I was. It was relaxing not to have any performance metrics to fret about. Enjoy cruising along, enjoy observing and enjoy the satisfaction of getting through a bad patch when you might be tempted to quit. Racing in this way can indeed be a form of mental relaxation.

Since my desert initiation into ultra-running, I have now upgraded to a GPS watch. I activate the timer to record time and distance but generally don't look at it whilst running. A stage further is that on some days, particularly when my enthusiasm to train is at a low ebb, I leave the watch at home. You miss out on gathering the statistics but enjoy the mental release of going fast, or slow, or stopping to admire the view, or whatever else takes your fancy.

Relaxation in the desert was particularly satisfying after a long hot day. The social interaction and comradeship of our tent of eight people was tremendous. We had not met before arriving at the race, but after a couple of days we saw ourselves as a team. The fact that we all finished is testament to team cohesion, which kept everyone going through some very hard stages. One of our number worked as a professional chef but was also an amateur stand-up comic. He had an endless supply of gags to kept us in good spirits. It was impressive how good he was at engaging with his audience. Soon after the end of each stage, the tent was blue with his humour. When the only female runner in our tent finished and returned to the tent, he would switch to less racy material. He was enjoying the escape of putting on his stand-up comic hat; and we enjoyed the escape of the free entertainment. I sometimes wonder what aspect of our time together have become gags in his stand-up routine.

Another member of MDS tent 119 was ex-Army and had many of the characteristics of a tank. I use that word in the most positive way possible, as he was of sturdy build and would persevere through whatever difficulties he encountered. He was slow but also unstoppable. His feet were shredded and his back rubbed raw from his backpack. Each night his feet would need strapping up to get through the next day. On the longest stage he came into the tent last of us, not long before the cut-off time. He must have been hurting but did not once complain. At the opposite end of the performance scale, the first person back each day was a fast runner who travelled exceedingly light. He chose not to carry a cooker so each evening he ate his freeze-dried meal cold. For my part that was a deprivation too far. As I mentioned previously, I carried a lightweight stove and would heat enough water to hydrate a hot meal and make a brew. Later in the week I donated my brew water so he could have a hot meal. Strictly, in a race of total self-sufficiency, we were breaking race rules, but I couldn't watch him suffer another cold sachet of goop. Overall, desert evenings in the company of such an eclectic group of people were more relaxing than any evening down the pub.

It is easy to accept that to relax after a long run feels good, if only because the punishment is over. If you are a dedicated runner, you will know that the running itself can also be relaxing. For non-runners, it might be easier to understand by a comparison with cycling. I no longer enjoy cycling on public roads after I was hit by a car travelling at high speed. Recovery from my injuries, which included a broken back, took over a year. I still enjoy riding my static bike, firmly rooted to one spot in the garage. I plan my cycling by looking at the radio schedule and choosing an interesting programme. I then cycle and listen to the programme at the same time. Of course, it would be relaxing to sit in a chair and enjoy the same radio programme, but this can be enhanced by concurrent cycling – provided the pace feels comfortable. My conscious mind is focussed on the radio programme, whilst my legs are spinning the pedals on autopilot. The same detached relaxed movement is possible when you run, but it takes time and cumulative miles to reach a level of running where this is possible.

The problem that everyone encounters is that the occasional run hurts. If you don't run regularly, running is not relaxing. It is physically tiring and has a high impact on the joints. When you run regularly over long distances, you learn to cruise, allowing your legs to stride on autopilot with your mind any place you choose to take it. For the regular runner, a long run can be just as relaxing as a snooze on the sofa. Of course, you can have the best of both, if after a long run and something to eat, you also have a snooze on the sofa.

Many people, especially older people, are trapped in an inactivity downward spiral. The mindset which can take hold is that I don't run and if I do, it hurts. This is enough to justify not running, reinforcing the spiral of decline. To escape, you must break the cycle. This requires the courage to force yourself to run, to endure the discomfort, until you learn to cruise, and until it becomes an enjoyable activity. How long this takes depends on how long you have been caught in the activity down spiral. This requires patience because it is important that you ease into it. Again, good general guidance is not to increase your mileage by more than 10 per cent per week. When you decide to ramp up, be honest about the starting point. Don't start with the mileage you would like to be doing, but with the mileage you are *actually* doing. If this is zero, then you are mathematically snookered. Ten per cent of nothing is nothing. In this case, you need to spend a week running short distances well within your capability. Whatever you achieve in that first week can be your baseline.

I have three enduring pictures in my mind which illustrates the relaxation of ultra-running. One was recorded on the third and final day of a multi-day ultra race along the Ridgeway in Southern England. That day was structured in reverse order, beginning with a mass start followed later by the runners who were leading after the first two days. These fast runners were set off according to their accumulated time. This ensured that the first person over the finishing line on the final day was the winner of the whole multi-day stage race. Of course, I was in the mass start of those not in contention for the top places. As the day progressed, I was overtaken by the fast runners, the last of whom was the man who was leading the three-day race. The mental video clip which stays with me is the way he seemed to be bouncy – effortless, relaxed and fast. It reminded me of the Winnie the Pooh character Tigger, springing along without a care in the world feeling just Grrreat! Meanwhile I was not feeling bouncy and appreciated that he took the time to offer me some words of encouragement as he bounced past. He was the epitome of a happy runner. At the prize-giving, he was humble and gave the impression of running simply for the fun of it.

My second strong memory comes from the double marathon stage of the Sahara race. It was a similar race format of a mass start with a later start time for the leading runners. As the day's race unfolded, the leading runners caught up with and overtook us slower runners. I remember with great clarity watching the top three runners come past together, two Moroccans and a British man. It was the way they ran which was so mesmerising: so smooth, so light on their feet, and so relaxed. I play back my mind's video sometimes when I am out running to try and copy their style. I think about long, loping strides using minimum effort and totally relaxed. I fail of course to get anywhere near the style captured in my memory but just thinking about it improves my gait and encourages a more relaxed style.

Over rough terrain, relaxed running is quite a challenge. The nature of the ground underfoot means you need to stay alert to trip hazards and unseen dips to be able to brace against unexpected. The natural response is to be tense and expend effort to ensure you are fully in control. Over long periods this is completely draining. The better method is to be fully relaxed but alert to taking back control in an instant. The combination of total physical relaxation whilst poised to catch a trip takes some learning.

My third mental video comes from the huge screen mounted in the centre of Chamonix showing the progress of the UTMB. The leader was coming off the mountains down towards the finish. I am not sure what technology was deployed, but I assume that the camera was on a drone flying above and behind the runner. The runner's style looked so effortless and easy as they descended the rocky path relying on gravity to do the work, each foot landing only fleetingly – just enough to retain control. This image is something I play back to myself on mountain descents. I cannot copy it towards the end when my legs have turned to jelly, but early in the race I too can bound down quite fast remaining alert to the possibility of a slippery or loose rock.

There is a knack to achieving the balancing act of relaxing whilst you are running. It isn't easy but I hope to have explained that it really is possible to run and relax. Such relaxation comes with a lot of mileage and experience. It also needs the confidence that the body has the strength and resilience to brace for the unexpected hazard, misstep or trip. It may not be possible to match the style of the elite runners, but with a relaxed attitude, well-cushioned shoes and an efficient stride, I believe that anyone can both run and relax.

In championing the case for ultra-running as relaxation, I admit that there is a simpler approach to relaxation, which is to back off from running. There is also space for this within the overall context of ultra-running.

CHAPTER 16

THE JOY OF NOT RUNNING

Not running can be even more fun than running.

To dedicated hard-core ultra-runners, not to run is unthinkable. They feel driven to run every day, with two runs a day not unusual. If you participate in ultra-running, you will meet such people. During one ultramarathon, a fellow runner struck up a conversation. He was keen to explain that in training he was running up to 250 km per week. He was clearly proud of this, and I replied with a positive response along the lines of being amazed that he could do such a huge mileage. I was indeed amazed; amazed that anyone could dedicate so much of their time to running. We were going along at a similar same pace and finished with much the same finish time. His huge training mileage seemed not to have achieved very much and left me wondering about the point of it.

Running can be an addiction in much the same way as alcohol. It is the ability to refrain from excess which is important. Feeling guilty because you are not out running is a sign that you may have a problem. Those who are afflicted with Compulsive Running Disorder (CRD) may not know it, as the compulsion to run slowly takes over their lives. It does not have the negative connotations of other compulsive behaviours, such as continually snacking on junk food, but not knowing when to desist from running is a psychological weakness that can be just as bad, if not worse. Extreme CRD could quite literally mean running yourself into an early grave. It would be so ironic to have the lean physique of an ultra-runner but to be outlived by your sedentary peers. Of course, as a runner you understand that living the life of a couch potato cannot be much fun. It could be, however, that their lazy indifference to activity could keep them alive, but in slowly increasing ill health, for years or decades longer that someone with extreme CRD. Running makes you feel great but overdoing it could be counterproductive. I am an avid proponent for using running to keep you firing on all cylinders, feeling great until your personal lights-out moment. That does not mean stressing your body to the point of premature failure.

On occasions, it is sensible to desist from running. Instead of fretting about not clocking up the miles, it is better to make the positive choice not to run. It should not be about failure to get out to run; it should be about succeeding in leaving your running shoes unused by the back door. On these days, not running should be a deliberate, positive choice rather than regarded as failure.

I am not ashamed to admit that I really enjoy not running. One implication of this statement is that I should run less. In fact, I could stop running and dedicate my leisure time to other activities. If you are not a running enthusiast, these words might chime with you. However, there is a flaw in such logic. It is only because you are running regularly over long distances that you can really appreciate the pleasure of choosing to take a break and not to run. Simply not running, taken out of context, would be no fun at all.

During the period preceding a big ultra race, it is particularly important to back off from running. This is different to preparing for shorter races, where you need to be fired up and bouncing along at a good lick from the starting gun. Ultra-running is a slow-burn sport in taking time to light the fire is just fine. Leading into an ultramarathon, one easy week before should suffice, with some simple exercises such as stretching and a few short jogs. For a long-distance ultra race, or multi-day ultra event, this period of very little running should be extended to two weeks. This is not just to ensure full physical recovery but also has a psychological benefit. By the time the race starts, you have been so deprived of running that you are itching to get back into it.

Another prime opportunity to enjoy not running is in the period after an ultra race. Sometimes this is because you are injured, or your feet are so cut up that you can't run. Assuming that you are capable of running, I believe it is important that you don't. Runners with CRD will argue you need to run again immediately the next day to help the recovery. This is like an alcoholic arguing that the best way to deal with a hangover is to have another drink. In an ultra race, your body will have taken a hammering, particularly if it was over mountainous terrain. It needs rest and recovery. This is a great time to enjoy, relax and feast in the glow of satisfaction of completing another monster challenge. My choice of words may seem like hyperbole, but ultra-running is about doing things in retirement that you would not believe are possible, until that is you cross the finishing line.

I find that I sleep particularly well during the period of post-race wind-down – except for the first night. When running over rough terrain, I spend so long concentrating on being ready to brace against a trip or slip, that for the night following the race my mind continues waking me up to avoid some imagined obstacle with my legs twitching. This does not apply to road races, where to fall over would be regarded as ridiculous. Running on smooth, flat tarmac requires little concentration, allowing the assumption that it is secure under foot, to such an extent that you can engage autopilot, with each stride the same. This repetitive motion is one of the reasons that road racing is so dull in comparison to trail running. After many hours tightly focussed on navigating rough trails, it can take a full 24 hours to reprogram your mind into truly relaxed mode. The days following participation in a race can include gentle exercise (not running), which might include a light session in the gym. At the end of the week, I feel recharged and wanting to bound back into running.

After a mega-ultra, I recommend a holiday. Selecting the next ultra-running challenge and holiday plans can be made in tandem. After all, if you are to put yourself through such a tough challenge, it makes sense to do it somewhere exotic and interesting. Double down on the fun to be had by staying on to explore the region and place. This message was driven home to me some years ago during my early career in the Army. I was selected to enter the inter-service marathon race held in the UK, starting and finishing at an RAF base. It was a midweek event, two laps of pancake-flat tarmac roads, and a field of about twenty runners. I do not remember a more depressing event, with nothing of interest in terms of scenery and only a handful of spectators. It was almost as if the event had been designed to be soul-destroying. In retirement, there is no need to accept such dull and demotivating races. You are in total control of when and where to race. You can choose the races you enter to go somewhere where you may not have been before, to explore new sights and discover unusual places.

A post-race holiday is not just about recovery but also a reward for having completed the race. It might also be the case that you have a long-suffering partner dragged along to spectate and support; the holiday can be a thank-you to them. They will get the bonus that for this particular holiday they will not be abandoned whilst you are out training. The focus can be on sight-seeing, coffee-drinking, cocktail-sipping, or whatever floats your boat. Hopefully the race will have been interesting, challenging, satisfying and perhaps even exciting. Pleasure is not a word which might come to mind; it is during the post-race holiday where this is to be found. Ultra-running can give a huge boost to the quality of your holiday enjoyment. Doing very little in pampered luxury may sound like fun but context is everything. Holidaymakers taking the same holiday, without an ultra race preceding it, are missing out. I remember post-race holidays which were tremendously relaxing and fun but taken in a different context would have been very dull indeed.

Running training that includes not running, may seem to be a contradiction in terms, but not necessarily. I remember a long and enjoyable day running in the Black Mountains, in south Wales. I started my GPS watch to log my session but did not look at it, nor use it to help navigate. I was using it simply to gather data I could reflect upon at the end of the day. I carried plenty of water and had packed a fresh wholemeal roll filled with cheese, cucumber and lettuce, one of my favourite combinations. At around halfway, at a high point with tremendous views, I put on my warm hat and windproof top, sat down and ate the sandwich slowly. This was so much more fun than monitoring pace and pushing on to record a decent time. This relatively short interlude was the highlight of the day.

Another example of the pleasure of not running came to mind when driving home from the Cape Wrath Ultra. The race had required navigating through the wilds of the Scottish Highlands for eight days, mostly off road in places no tourist would venture. After one last night under canvas at Cape Wrath, it had been a long four-hour coach journey back south through Scotland to the start at Fort William. This was a reminder, if one was needed, of just how far we had travelled using our steam in the preceding week. It was now time to reclaim my car, parked on a sports field by the start, and drive my battered body home. The beautiful Glencoe was on the route. The road goes through spectacular Scottish scenery on either side, with regular places to pull off the road to sight-see. The carparks were busy, allowing people to step out to take photos, perhaps walking 100 m or so to the best vantage point. Great pictures indeed, but the context is of a largely negative experience: driving, stopping, snapping and driving on. If you pause whilst ultra-running to take a picture, you can be completely absorbed within the scene, without a road or the sound of a car anywhere nearby. Stopping to snap such a view can be a moment of pure joy. The race clock keeps ticking, of course, but taking time to stop running, just for a minute, can be a welcome and invigorating respite. The memory of the moment can be lodged deep within your memory with the digital image file captured on your phone acting as the trigger, not of an interrupted car journey but of a moment of peace within the wilderness.

In this chapter, I write from the perspective of enjoying running, rather than pushing the pace and striving for the best race result. An ultra-runner, with whom I have shared several races, is much younger than me, and he is fast. He explained to me that he focussed on running as fast as the terrain would allow and his body would tolerate. This did not allow time or opportunity to observe the scenery or enjoy the location. To him, the focus was on the next stride, and the next, and the next. He would appear towards the top of the results list, but what a price to pay. He expressed regret that perhaps he was missing out, but he felt that he had to choose between racing and enjoying. I hope that when he is older, and age has slowed him down, rather than strive to retain a vestige of his former performance, he might join me in the simple enjoyment of participating.

CHAPTER 17

FUELLING THE ADDICTION

To finish is to win.

As you have read, the initial idea had taken hold to mark my sixtieth year by entering the Marathon des Sables (MDS). I intended this iconic week-long race across the Sahara to be a one-off special event. I had not anticipated that I would get drawn into the strange world of ultra-running. Like someone taking a single line of cocaine intending to stop at that, I had become hooked. Long, slow running had become a habit, a compulsion even. As you'll know from reading this far, some years after completing the MDS, I became fascinated by the even more extreme challenge of the Ultra Trail du Mont Blanc (UTMB). A much harder race, it involved 100 miles non-stop over steep mountainous terrain including running through two nights. To even get on the start list is an achievement, as you must complete qualifying races that demonstrate sufficient ultra-running experience. Unlike the MDS, which is accessible to almost anyone daft enough to give it a go, the full UTMB is restricted to only those fully inducted into the cohort of ultra-running oddballs. The UTMB cannot be undertaken lightly as an adventure; it requires a huge commitment and finishing cannot be assumed. If you do succeed in finishing, you are indeed a winner.

The original UTMB, based in Chamonix in the Alps, has been held every year since 2003, except for 2020 when it was cancelled due to the coronavirus pandemic. It falls at the end of August, usually coinciding with the UK late summer Bank Holiday. I qualified by completing the CCC 100 km race and the North Downs Way 100 mile race in southern England. I made the start line, no mean feat. Unfortunately for this, my first attempt, I was beaten by the enormity of the challenge and my difficulty at coping with running in mountainous terrain at night. This weakness would need addressing before making any further attempt. At the time, the embarrassment of not finishing had been a huge blow to both my ego and my confidence. I was being advised by well-meaning friends to be sensible, using the argument that no one my age should be attempting such a challenge. That was just the advice I needed. To be offered the excuse that old people shouldn't be doing this got me annoyed and fired up. I could not let this failure be the end my ultra-running career. I was determined that it would not end like this, although I had to admit that my first attempt at the UTMB did provide a dose of reality. There is indeed a limit to what an ageing body can endure.

This chapter focusses on returning to atone for my failure and finding out whether it was possible for an old man to tame the UTMB beast. This account helps to explain why ultra-running is so addictive.

As mentioned, the original UTMB event now has a series of spin-off events across the world. UTMB Nice is one of these, consisting of a series of races over one weekend. There is the short 20 km taster race; a 50 km ultramarathon, a tough 100 km mountain trail run, and the big one, a 100 mile mountain-running challenge that almost defies description. To call it extreme would be an understatement. After bombing out of the 100 mile UTMB Chamonix race, I managed to get an entry into the same-length UTMB Nice so that I could pitch myself again into the maelstrom of the big format race. The start is in the village of Auron in the Maritime Alps, with the route taking the runners through the mountains of the Mercantour National Park to the finish in Nice.

The finish line facilities were impressive – matching the status of the race – and erected on one of the Mediterranean's most impressive beachfronts, the Promenade des Anglais. The final 400 m was lined with barriers to hold back spectators, while a huge arch marked the finish line. Alongside this, there was a race village containing a wide range of temporary shops selling everything from running equipment and clothes to race food and information on other international ultra-running events, including the UTMB world series. These top-class facilities did justice to this major race, making you feel that you were part of something very special.

If the route had taken the easiest trails to navigate the 100 miles from high up in the mountains to the coast, that would have been a tough ultra race. If only that were so. The UTMB ethos does not include 'easy'. The route ticked off a whole series of high mountain passes on the way. It seems to have been designed to take the hardest possible route, which I am sure is the organizers' intention as they vie for it to be as hard, or harder, than the original UTMB. In summary, the UTMB Nice is not just tough, it is a cruel beast of a mountain ultramarathon.

I knew before I started that finishing was not a given. A friend of mine didn't help before the race by telling me about a hiking holiday with friends in the same mountain range. He had explained that over a week they had hiked part of the route, doing up to 15 km each day on their way to the next night's accommodation. Their suitcases had been transported for them to the target hotel, so they needed to carry only a day pack. There had been an excellent dinner, a good night's sleep and a full breakfast before tackling the next day's route. That sounded relaxed and great fun. He went on to explain, not entirely encouragingly, that he couldn't envisage that the daily hikes could have been much longer than 15 km because the terrain had been so rugged and steep. He questioned the wisdom of entering a race requiring participants to tackle the Maritime Alps in one hit without a break and no sleep. This was extreme beyond extreme; tough beyond tough; and brutal to an extent that is hard to comprehend – unless you have tried it. My friend was totally unsupportive of my aspirations, advising that it would be impossible – at my age. He was unaware that his well-meant advice was like showing a red flag to a bull. When anyone says to me 'not at your age', it makes me angry. I felt like screaming back 'No!' but I held my tongue and resolved that I would prove him wrong and give it a go.

That said, the closer I got to setting off to Nice, entering the UTMB did indeed start to look like attempting the impossible. As the start day approached, my trepidation had mounted and my resolve had been tested severely. I examined any tiny niggle as a sign that I might be injured. My subconscious seemed to be looking for a valid reason to withdraw. Of course, during the race itself, all sorts of valid reasons to withdraw arose and needed to be faced down, but on the start line I had been fit, well and devoid of a good excuse.

Two full nights and the best part of two days later, eventually, the pain was over. Having attempted the impossible, all I wanted was a place to crash out. I wanted to get to my hotel room but the route towards a hot shower and a bed with crisp clean sheets meant going through the UTMB race village and its shop: in fact, you couldn't avoid it. The latter's displays would not be out of place in any up-market department store, with prices to match. The clothes racks, shelves and display podiums were designed to persuade you to make a purchase. For those who did manage to finish, this is where a wide range of apparel could be purchased to wear with pride, championing their achievement. The prices of the branded garments were indeed high but were dirt cheap in comparison to the personal price extracted if you had completed the full race.

I was walking slowly, completely on empty. I needed a break, sat down on the edge of a display podium amongst the pristine new garments and glitzy displays. I was not inclined to start browsing. I had money hidden deep inside my race backpack in a waterproof pouch (as required by the race rules in case of getting lost and needed to pay for transport or assistance). I was not in a mood to consider digging out my emergency cash stash. I was enjoying the respite of not going anywhere. My legs did not want to hold me standing up, let alone allow me to walk. My mental and physical reserves were completely depleted. I had been running on empty throughout the past night. I slumped forward with my head down, noticing the filthy shorts, socks and shoes. It looked like I had been wading in mud, which was not far off the truth. A storm had rolled in during the first night making the paths muddy and the rocky parts slippery. The treacherous conditions abated in the latter stages of the race and the weather had been kinder, allowing me to at least dry out. My legs were now caked in dried mud and blood from the numerous bangs and scrapes. I wondered if the dark stain on my running shoe was fresh blood oozing out, but I could not be sure. In my determination to press on, I had not taken off my shoes to check my feet since taking a longer pause at one of the aid stations late in the afternoon of the second day.

Sitting in this retail space, with my head in my hands, tears came to my eyes. I am not a demonstrative person so I was surprised to find myself shaking gently with emotion. I received a tap on my shoulder. I lifted my head to meet the searching gaze of a young woman wearing a T-shirt bearing the UTMB logo. I tried to hide my tears as she asked if I was okay. I must have looked a pathetic sight. It was good of her to check up on me, and I suspected she would also rather I was not making a mess of her retail space. I reflected before replying. An honest reply might see me taken away to the medical tent. I wanted to be in my hotel room, not on a stretcher with a drip in my arm.

The sales assistant was waiting for my reply. I wanted to compose myself and not show how weak and emotional I was. Finally, I explained that I was sitting down here in her shop involuntarily, because of extreme tiredness. I was bombed out, sore, and happy not to be running anymore. Yet I was also, in fact ecstatic, despite appearances. The tears I tried to hide were not tears brought on by failure but tears of joy. I had indeed finished. I had never felt so emotional at the end of a race event. This was a life-affirming totally mad escapade. It was a realignment of what I believed was possible. A re-set of expectations. I thanked her for her concern and explained that I would get up shortly and move on. At that moment, I was not perhaps the best advertisement for the UTMB. If this was what the race does to participants, it would be reasonable to wonder why anyone would bother to enter.

The chilling example comes to mind of heroin addicts slumped in the street, looking terrible but having just injected, feeling on an emotional high. To an onlooker, an addict after a fix and an ultra-runner at the end of an extreme race may look similar, but there is one important difference. Heroin surging through your veins makes you feel good (so I am told) but destroys your long-term health. The endorphins from ultra-running provide a high (as I know well) and keeps you in blooming good health. The combination of long slow running and the accompanying emotional high leads to improved health over the long-term, even though it can be so shattering in the short-term. Ultra-running may indeed be an addiction, but one to embrace.

I did stand up and move on, evicted like a tramp who had fallen asleep in an up-market boutique. I noted that I would return later to buy a full set of clothes, bearing the race logo, to wear with pride. A magic carpet to whisk me direct the hotel would have been welcome. More realistically, I thought that one more kilometre (after so many) should hardly matter. I was walking with more confidence now. I didn't care who saw me. Wandering the streets of the cosmopolitan city of Nice bedraggled and filthy would normally single a person out as a vagrant and put one at possible risk of arrest. As I was still displaying my race number, I hoped that the stares I received were of admiration, not pity.

I walked, or more accurately shuffled, west along the Promenade des Anglais towards my hotel two blocks back from the coast. I didn't want the expense of paying for a sea view, but I did want to be a short walk from the finish. Hotels in central Nice do not come cheap but the Hôtel de France fitted my needs and was good value.

***

For the night before the race, I had stayed in the commercial district of Nice in the cheapest room I could find. It lived up to my low expectations. The hotel didn't look like a hotel at all; it was more like a building site. The stairwell was littered with building detritus and when I had arrived in the afternoon, the chance of a siesta was lost to the sound of power saws, drills and hammering. The building was under refurbishment, but when the working day was over it was quiet, and I had slept well. In another context, this hotel would seem like hitting rock bottom – a tiny room with a small single bed. In the context of spending the next two nights on my feet, running without a break and no sleep, the hotel seemed like pure luxury. That is one of the joys of ultra-running; to be deprived of basic comforts for long periods means that you really appreciate the simple pleasures of comfortable modern living. If you don't ultra-run, you might take your circumstances for granted and not enjoy the simple pleasure of being warm, safe and able to snooze as you wish. The words I have just written describe the life of a care-home resident, and not particularly riveting. When such activity is interspersed with ultra-running, such simple comforts become something to really savour and enjoy.

The day of the race had begun with a walk from my cheap accommodation wearing my running clothes and race backpack that contained all the mandatory safety equipment: warm long-sleeve top, warm hat, gloves, waterproof hooded jacket, waterproof over trousers, emergency bivvy bag, two head torches with spare batteries, emergency rations, medical kit, and a fully charged phone with additional external battery. That is all I would need for the next forty-eight hours. In addition, I was wheeling a suitcase with my normal clothes, wash bag, and general stuff for after the race. I stopped in a streetside café for coffee and a croissant. The hotel I had just left did not offer breakfast and I didn't want much in any case. Caffeine and carbs would be just fine. I arrived at Hôtel de France thinking that on another occasion this would be a comfy base from which to spend the weekend pottering around and exploring the sights of Nice. It was with a hint of regret that I explained that my reservation was for two days hence and all I wanted for now was to drop off my suitcase in advance. The logic I had employed when making the reservation was that there was no point in holding, and paying for, a hotel room whilst I was in the mountains. Not only was this a cost-effective solution; it was also a further incentive to complete the race. If I had dropped out prematurely, I had no accommodation to go to. I was given a paper docket with a number on it and my suitcase was taken away behind reception. I left through the front door of the hotel with the hotel reception staff smiling and wishing me luck. What they were really thinking I couldn't tell. I hoped that the smiles were of admiration but perhaps it was stifled laughter of amusement. For my own mindset, I was at a low point of self-doubt.

Walking through the streets of Nice, to where buses were waiting to take race participants to the start, I perked up, looking forward to the race with both nervousness and excitement. As I got to the rendezvous; more people converged dressed similarly with compact ultra-racing backpacks. I started to feel like a member of the fraternity of mountain ultra-runners. I hope I looked the part; but I couldn't eliminate the sense of imposter syndrome. I had not completed such a huge race before. Perhaps I would be a fraud who would start and complete the first day before exiting ignominiously.

We boarded the bus, some people in pairs or joking around in groups, and some like me as lone wolves. I overheard many stories and discussions about other races and people's training. I didn't want to engage. My own preparations were not impressive, and my previous experience limited. I gazed out of the window as the bus picked its way through the suburbs of Nice, heading north 100 miles to the start. It seemed like an awfully long bus ride. Bear in mind that the bus took the easiest possible most direct available route. Low gear was needed to make progress on the steepest bits as we climbed into the remote mountains. Sitting riding the bus was easy. I reflected on how I could possibly retrace the same journey on foot under my own steam; and it worried me. Not wanting to be too graphic in this account, I would need to make use of the rest facilities when the bus arrived. Off to the side were beautiful mountain vistas requiring peering upwards to observe the tops. Up there along the ridges and over the mountain passes was our route back to Nice. The bus ride had been long, tortuous, and somewhat disconcerting; the race route would be even more so.

Finally, we arrived in the small mountain village of Auron late morning. I walked off the bus into fine warm late September weather carrying my race backpack. I reflected on a full range of emergency equipment I was required to carry, as specified in the race rules. This is subject to spot checks at the start and along the route with risk of disqualification if something was found to be missing. In such good weather the list of mandatory equipment seemed over the top. If the weather had stayed the same, much of this kit would have remained in the pack throughout the race. That was not to be; when we were caught in a storm, I was glad to have enough to survive and get me through. I also carried two drop bags to hand into the race organizers at the start. These would be transported to the aid stations in Saint-Sauveur (63 km) and Levens (114 km) along the route. The chance to change to clean dry socks, and eat and drink my own selected supplies, would be welcome. The second drop bag also included a blister-repair kit of scalpel, antiseptic and bandages to repair the inevitable damage to my feet. I had finally learnt the lessons of how to be properly prepared by expecting the worst.

It was still a couple of hours until the 13:00 start time. In my enthusiasm when registering, I had booked a place on one of the first buses. The mountain village was idyllic, and we were blessed with warm sunshine. I found an outdoor table at a café and ordered a coffee and my second croissant of the day. This really felt like a great interlude and wonderful way to count down to the start. My enjoyment was brought into even sharper focus (and tinged with foreboding) knowing that a storm was rolling in, which would hit during our first night in the mountains. To keep my seat at the café, I had yet another coffee. As I would be awake for the next two nights, I assumed that extra caffeine would do no harm.

***

Early in the morning two days later, I was there at the finish. I had traversed from a mountain village bathed in warm sunshine to the Mediterranean coast as the sun was again rising. The forty hours between these two delightful locations could be described as both the best and worst of mountain trail running. The best was when the weather lifted allowing views of spectacular scenery. The worst was in a raging storm at night on slippery and dangerous terrain with sheer drops hidden by the dark.

Arriving again at the Hôtel de France, my mind was focussed on the immediate priorities of shower, food and sleep, preferably in that order. The hotel staff were welcoming and handed me my room key. I had misplaced or lost the paper docket to reclaim my suitcase, but they remembered me and retrieved my bag from behind reception. When staying in hotels, I invariably use the stairs as the healthy option; this time, I took the lift. Arriving in the room, the bed looked so inviting that I could have crashed out on the spot. I looked from the pristine bedspread to my filthy body and thought better of it.

How to clean myself up without trashing the room was a puzzle and I was in no mood for complex solutions. Leaving my suitcase by the door, I went into the walk-in shower wearing all my running gear, including shoes and backpack. I stood under the water, allowing the filth to wash off. I then started to undress. My socks were particularly difficult to remove. It was not just the fact that they seemed stuck to my feet by congealed blood, but simply the act of bending down to remove them was beyond me. I sat on the shower floor to peel off my socks. After showering myself, I picked out each item from the pile of dirty rags on the shower floor, rinsed them and squeezed out the water. They were still filthy, but the loose mud and detritus was now removed. I used every protruding item in the bathroom to hang everything up. What had been a swish bathroom now looked like a back-street poor-quality laundry.

The next task was to examine myself. Fresh blood was dripping from hands that had been injured when arresting a fall in the mountains. The deep cuts had reopened as I cleaned the wounds. I could see that my big toenails were coming adrift, but they were attached for now. All in all, I was surprisingly well. Drying myself, I had tried not to get blood on the hotel towels, but I failed as there were too many minor injuries to avoid: sorry, hotel staff. Despite my good intentions, the bathroom was a mess. At least the main room had been spared.

The bed was again the centre of my attention, looking comfortable and inviting. I worried that if I lay down, I would be out for the count. I needed food and breakfast was downstairs. I took the lift. Entering the breakfast room, it was a pleasure not to have to grab a quick snack and run on. I could fill my plate and sit and eat, and then repeat, and repeat again. One of the highlights of ultra-running is eating to recover, sometimes in quite outrageous quantities, knowing that hours later you will again be ravenously hungry. Oddly, on this occasion, I was so depleted and run down that I had soon had enough. It was as if even the effort of eating was too much.

Feeling clean, well fed and a bit stronger, I went back to my room via the stairs. I regretted my decision as soon as I climbed the first one. I did not need more practice at ascending. Finally, I was in a fit state to use the bed. After no sleep for two days, I assumed that I would sleep like a log, so I set an alarm. I wanted a short nap and then get up to watch the closing prize ceremony and applaud the last runners coming in before the cut-off time of 13:00. It was Sunday morning, and the race had started middle of the day on Friday. I reflected on whether I would rather have spent the previous couple of days exploring

Nice and its cafes or 100 miles of mountain trails without sleep. I had made the right choice, but now was the time to relax, and catch up on sleep.

I did indeed drop off to sleep almost immediately; although just as quickly, I woke up with a start. My legs were twitching. The instinct to keep moving and stay upright had not turned off. I woke up again, feeling that I had just caught myself before falling. Maybe I slept a little, but I would not get a good night's sleep until that evening. Mentally, winding down from such focussed intense activity takes time.

My mind was avoiding reflecting over much on the previous two days. My mental defence mechanisms were already starting to blank out some of it. Retaining the good memories and archiving the bad ones is my approach to staying sane – I learnt that in my time in the military. I think that the opposite approach of dwelling on bad memories undermines mental health. My experience leads me to push back strongly against the experts who recommend reliving and recounting bad experiences. In my opinion, it's best to put them aside. Don't forget them, but do not dwell on them; what is done is done. On the positive side, one recent pleasant memory also came back to me.

***

The final aid station before the finish was Plateau Saint Michel, 154 km into the race; the more important statistic was that it was 10 km from the finish. To complete the race was now inevitable: I could walk all the way to the end and still be within the cut-off time. The huge weight of lingering doubt that had been my companion throughout the event had lifted. I arrived at the aid station as dawn was breaking, always a psychological lift. The sustenance laid out included pieces of banana, chocolate and other high-energy foods. I selected hot coffee and a slice of cake.

At most previous aid stations I had stayed on my feet, grabbed something quickly and gone on my way. At this ultimate aid station, I felt able to relax a little. I had long since given up pushing for a fast time. I was not even looking at my phone using the app that would show live race positions and time splits – if I wanted to see them. I wasn't bothered; the time was irrelevant now. My only objective was to finish. Why not enjoy the moment? There was a line of chairs out in the open air off to the side. I plonked myself down and proceeded to sip the coffee, munch the cake and watched the sun creep up over the horizon. Competitors arrived, fuelled up and moved on. From their athletic manner, I assumed that most of these people were coming towards the completion of one of the shorter events with later departure times and start locations closer to Nice. This final stretch was common to all routes. The 164 km entrants were easy to spot: gaunt, tired and suffering. I needed that moment of calm, enjoying coffee outside in the cool of the early dawn of what would later be a warm summer day. I was not to know that during the twenty minutes or so that I spent there, another person in my age group was hunting me down. There are age-group listings within the main event, a race within a race, with people taking pride in their position relative to others. Somewhere behind me, a French runner was racing to improve his position in the over-60 category.

Finally, I had stood up to get moving again. Any bounce that my legs once had, was gone. I walked much of that final 10 km, with periods where I lifted my pace to a slow shuffling run. I entered the outskirts of Nice with the route picking off a few more hills on the way. Even for this last section the route was planned to be as tough as the terrain could provide.

The final kilometres followed the coastal route from the East. As I rounded the harbour of Port Lympia, I was entering one of the tourist areas of Nice. A retired British couple chose to walk beside me. They explained that when they realised that the UTMB was in town, they had been following it online; in particular, they had been following me, so they said. I felt honoured. I knew my wife would look at the live feed to check if I was still alive, but the idea that anyone else could be interested gave me a bit of a lift. Perhaps they were just being kind.

As the finish line approached, there was a funnel of barriers keeping back crowds of spectators with the finishing banner visible further along the Promenade des Anglais. My pride told me that I should try to run this one last kilometre. I said my farewell to my supporters and broke into a run, trying to look like an athlete. The crowds were denser the nearer I got to the finish line and the applause was tremendous. I was not listening to the content of the race commentary, but it added to the feeling that this a special occasion. How good, I thought, that even those arriving well after the leaders were getting such a warm reception.

After crossing the line, I was interviewed and my words broadcast over the public address system. Again, I thought how good it was that ordinary runners like me were being allowed their moment of glory. I don't remember what I said, but I assumed I lied. I would have said something appropriate such as how much I had enjoyed it.

Having lifted myself up to match the image of an ultra-runner for the final kilometre and continuing to hold my composure to answer the interviewer's questions, I started to wilt. Beyond the finish, I had shuffled past the medical support facilities without being pulled aside for special attention. I must have looked as if I was okay. As I mentioned earlier, the way out was funnelled through the UTMB merchandise tent. It was there that I had semi-collapsed and sat with my head in my hands, emotional, and feeling unable to go another step.

***

By midday, I had found my way back along the Promenade des Anglais, strolling slowly in the warm sunshine, to return to the finish area. Stragglers were still coming in. For them, the challenge was to finish inside the cut-off time. Each participant was running their own race, against their own targets and expectations. To come first would of course be extraordinary, but to complete the event within the cut-off time is also to win. Both the runner who was first over the line and the back markers are all winners, each in their own way. I felt like a winner; and it felt good. Physically, I was completely stuffed, wiped out, thumped, hammered, drained and any other word that describes the weakest state possible and still be breathing. Emotionally, I was flying high as a bird, soaring above the immediacy of the soreness and pain.

I was wearing my crisp clean race T-shirt with pride and the finishing medal around my neck. I now understood the attraction of ultra-running. It is not about winning; it is about challenging yourself to tackle something seemingly impossible and to come out on top. To finish is to win.

The prize-giving would soon start, and I took up position to watch the proceedings. I wanted to see the people who were on the podium, to see what sort of people they were, and whether they too looked wiped out. The race winners were announced first, with one of them leaping up onto the podium as if their legs had already recovered. I assume this was more bravado than reality, but it was impressive. Pictures were taken of the top men and women athletes before moving onto the age-group prizes. These were awarded in reverse order starting with the younger runners. As each award was made, the group of winners expanded filling the now crowded stage. I looked on at this impressive group of people, in admiration that they looked so well, when I was still feeling totally pole-axed.

Finally, it came to the awards for my age group of men over sixty. There were prizes for first and second. A French name was announced. Out of the watching crowd of spectators, a man walked forward and climbed the steps onto the podium wearing running shorts which showed thin sinewy tightly muscled legs. He looked every bit a top-class ultra-runner. I reflected that he was a living example that ultra-running in old age is good for you. Then my name was announced over the public address system. This was not something I had expected. As I had struggled to keep going through that second night, I had given up any lingering dreams of being on the podium at the finish. I was oblivious to the fact that as people succumbed to the extreme tiredness and pain, many had dropped out. Those left in my age group had been thinning out as the race had progressed. I didn't know (or bother to care) that I was still in contention for the age-group award. As the second dawn had broken, I had lingered at the final aid station enjoying the sun rise and savouring an extended moment of supreme satisfaction. I could relax, being sure of completing the final stretch to the finish well inside the cut-off time.

Unknown to me, I was in fact in the lead, not of the race of course, but of my sub-category. I was being called to the podium as the over-60 male winner. I picked my way forward through the crowd, forcing my pummelled legs to stride confidently, wanting to look like I deserved the honour. This was why I had been interviewed at the finish, why the tourists had been following my progress, and my reward for pushing hard and holding it together through the storm on that first night. I had indeed nearly been overhauled through the second night. If I had known that I was still in the race, I may not have enjoyed the last 10 km as much, wanting to keep up the pace. If my lazy finish had been even slightly slower, I would have lost. The results showed that the Frenchman had finished three minutes behind me. My decision to run the last kilometre had been fortunate. This was out of simple pride, not because I thought there was any chance of the age-group prize. In my mind I had been a winner simply by completing the event. To find that I was also first in my age group was a wonderful bonus. Of course, being the first old man in an ultra-mountain trail event is of no significance to anyone – except to me.

Whilst on the winners' stage, I looked around at the spectators with thoughts that this was surreal and for me a beautiful moment. I looked around at my fellow winners, in particular I took a searching look at the old man standing beside me who had been second. This man had been hunting me down and had come close to pipping me on the line. I opened a conversation, wanting to know if he had known that I was just in front. Had he been conscious of racing me to the line? Initially, he did not respond to my English, so I switched to French. The chance of a deep conversation was limited by my linguistic ability, but we shared a few brief thoughts. The gist of our short conversation was agreement that the race had been extremely hard and a great experience. I couldn't be sure whether these were his true thoughts, or like me, he may have been saying what seemed right for the occasion. In answer to my question as to whether he would be back for another attempt, his response was immediate. He spoke an emphatic 'Non!' So, we were both in the same place, where the pain is so recent and so raw that you never, ever, want to repeat it.

Usually, time is great healer and after a while your reflections of an event, particularly one as tough and as satisfying as the UTMB, slowly evolve from never-ever-again to the possibility of coming back for more. I admit to being an addict for ultra-running, and addicts struggle to stay clean, so what comes next? At the time of writing this book, I reflect that now could be a good time to finish on a high. Although I intend to continue ultra-running until the day I drop, I should hold back from entering any more of the extreme races. It would not be sensible to go back for another dose of the full UTMB. The problem is that ultra-running does not do sensible …

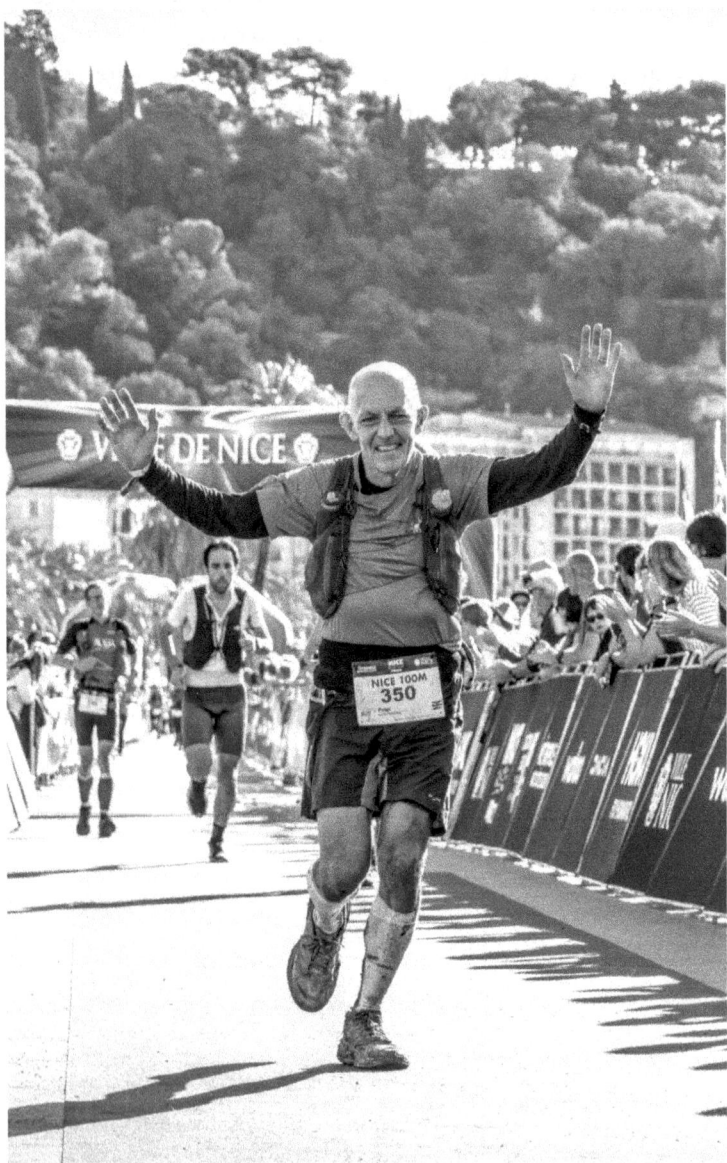

Crossing the finish line at Nice Côte d'Azur by UTMB® 2022

EPILOGUE

The attraction of taking up ultra-running is not because it is easy, but because it is hard. There is no need to be a speedy athlete to join this wonderful (if nutty) fraternity. You just need to want to give it a go and have the determination to get started. Injury and ill health can always get in the way, of course, but once you have entered the world of ultra-running, such slow sustained activity is the best medicine you can take. As protection against chronic medical conditions, it is hard to beat. Instead of sitting around asking the doctor to treat your symptoms and ailments, give your body the very best chance to heal itself. I am not a medical professional, so my words should be read with caution, but, in my view, no one should be considered too old or infirm to become an ultra-runner. It is true that the transition from couch potato to long-distance runner is hard – really hard. Not everyone will make it through, but the destination is worth the pain. When the fascination with ultra-running takes hold, it takes over. Instead of running because you feel you should, you run because you want to. Once you are an ultra-runner, sitting still for long periods is not easy. I accept that ultra-running may be regarded by some as compulsion, but one to be embraced. Ultra-running comes with both positives and negatives. On the positive side, is renewed health and vitality; on the negative side, for older people, is the risk that running might be your finale. Ultra-running in old age is to live life to the full, until the day you drop.

As I investigate new and interesting ultra-races, I now avoid events where the organizers require a medical certificate, as my doctor has become increasingly reluctant to sign off for the more extreme races. I suspect he does not want to be responsible in case one day, I do not make it through. My manuscript editor has reminded me that I should not be advising ignoring medical advice. Quite so, my advice is to do only that which your doctor will support. The fact that I ignore my own advice is for me alone. I feel in the peak of health, which is exactly the point. I am fit and feel just great, continuing to train regularly and undertake ultra-marathons. It is my contention that it is because I participate in ultramarathons that I continue to feel on top form. If I stop, I feel certain that I will enter the downward spiral of age-related ill health. If I carry on, I am confident of staying fit and well for the rest of my life, be it short or long.

To enter ultra-running events is to put yourself well outside your comfort zone. To undertake such severe challenges, tinged with uncertainty, is a great way to spice up your retirement. Running across the Sahara or circumnavigating 100 miles of mountain trails around Mont Blanc non-stop may be at the extreme end of the ultra-running scale and not for everyone, but why not aim high, run long, and take on the challenge? Remember that to finish is to win; the opponent is your own limits not other runners.